THE JOHNS HOPKINS REVIEW OF GYNECOLOGY & OBSTETRICS

THE JOHNS HOPKINS REVIEW OF GYNECOLOGY & OBSTETRICS

Department of Gynecology and Obstetrics
The Johns Hopkins University School of Medicine
Baltimore, Maryland

EDITORS

BRANDON J. BANKOWSKI, MD
Department of Gynecology and Obstetrics
The Johns Hopkins University School of Medicine
Baltimore, Maryland

AMY E. HEARNE, MD
Department of Gynecology and Obstetrics
The Johns Hopkins University School of Medicine
Baltimore, Maryland

EDWARD E. WALLACH, MD
Department of Gynecology and Obstetrics
The Johns Hopkins University School of Medicine
Baltimore, Maryland

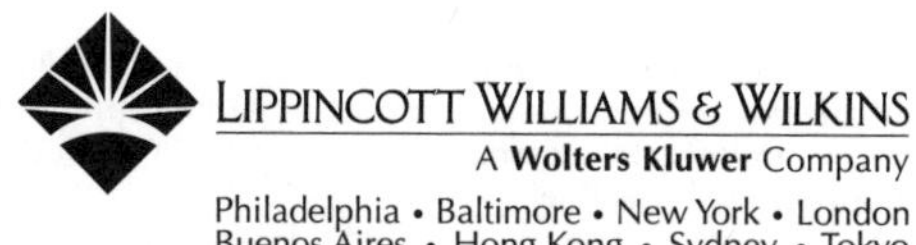

Acquisitions Editor: Ruth Weinburg
Developmental Editor: Julia Seto
Production Editor: Bridgett Dougherty
Manufacturing Manager: Ben Rivera
Marketing Manager: Sarah Bodison
Compositor: TechBooks
Printer: R.R. Donnelley—Crawfordsville

530 Walnut Street
Philadelphia, PA 19106 USA
LWW.com

Printed in the USA

Library of Congress Cataloging-in-Publication Data

The Johns Hopkins review of obstetrics & gynecology / Department of Gynecology and Obstetrics, the Johns Hopkins University School of Medicine; editors, Brandon J. Bankowski, Amy E. Hearne, Edward E. Wallach.
p. ; cm.
Includes index.
ISBN 0-7817-5173-x (pbk.)
1. Obstetrics—Examinations, questions, etc. 2. Gynecology—Examinations, questions, etc. I. Title: Review of obstetrics & gynecology. II. Bankowski, Brandon J. III. Hearne, Amy E. IV. Wallach, Edward E., 1933– V. Johns Hopkins University. Dept. of Gynecology and Obstetrics.
[DNLM: 1. Genital Diseases, Female—Problems and Exercises. 2. Genitalia, Female—physiology—Problems and Exercises. 3. Gynecology—methods—Problems and Exercises. 4. Obstetrics—methods—Problems and Exercises. 5. Pregnancy—physiology—Problems and Exercises. 6. Pregnancy Complications—Problems and Exercises. WP 18.2 J65 2004]
RG111.J635 2004
618′.076—dc22

2004015937

---

10 9 8 7 6 5 4 3 2 1

Contents

Contributors

Abimbola Aina MD
Department of Gynecology and Obstetrics
The Johns Hopkins University School of Medicine
Baltimore, Maryland

Carolyn Alexander MD
Department of Gynecology and Obstetrics
The Johns Hopkins University School of Medicine
Baltimore, Maryland

Brandon Bankowski MD
Department of Gynecology and Obstetrics
The Johns Hopkins University School of Medicine
Baltimore, Maryland

Songhai Barclift MD
Department of Gynecology and Obstetrics
The Johns Hopkins University School of Medicine
Baltimore, Maryland

Kim Bernard MD
Department of Gynecology and Obstetrics
The Johns Hopkins University School of Medicine
Baltimore, Maryland

Karin Blakemore MD
Department of Gynecology and Obstetrics
The Johns Hopkins University School of Medicine
Baltimore, Maryland

Betty Chou MD
Department of Gynecology and Obstetrics
The Johns Hopkins University School of Medicine
Baltimore, Maryland

Alice Chung MD
Department of Gynecology and Obstetrics
The Johns Hopkins University School of Medicine
Baltimore, Maryland

Jude Crino MD
Department of Gynecology and Obstetrics
The Johns Hopkins University School of Medicine
Baltimore, Maryland

Julia Cron MD
Department of Gynecology and Obstetrics
The Johns Hopkins University School of Medicine
Baltimore, Maryland

Janice Falls MD
Department of Gynecology and Obstetrics
The Johns Hopkins University School of Medicine
Baltimore, Maryland

Kim Fortner MD
Department of Gynecology and Obstetrics
The Johns Hopkins University School of Medicine
Baltimore, Maryland

Ruchi Garg MD
Department of Gynecology and Obstetrics
The Johns Hopkins University School of Medicine
Baltimore, Maryland

Dana Gossett MD
Department of Gynecology and Obstetrics
The Johns Hopkins University School of Medicine
Baltimore, Maryland

Ernest Graham MD
Department of Gynecology and Obstetrics
The Johns Hopkins University School of Medicine
Baltimore, Maryland

Edith Gurewitsch MD
Department of Gynecology and Obstetrics
The Johns Hopkins University School of Medicine
Baltimore, Maryland

Amy Hearne MD
Department of Gynecology and Obstetrics
The Johns Hopkins University School of Medicine
Baltimore, Maryland

Cynthia Holcroft MD
Department of Gynecology and Obstetrics
The Johns Hopkins University School of Medicine
Baltimore, Maryland

Julie Huh MD
Department of Gynecology and Obstetrics
The Johns Hopkins University School of Medicine
Baltimore, Maryland

Julie Jolin MD
Department of Gynecology and Obstetrics
The Johns Hopkins University School of Medicine
Baltimore, Maryland

Amer Karam MD
Department of Gynecology and Obstetrics
The Johns Hopkins University School of Medicine
Baltimore, Maryland

Lisa Kolp MD
Department of Gynecology and Obstetrics
The Johns Hopkins University School of Medicine
Baltimore, Maryland

Shari Lawson MD
Department of Gynecology and Obstetrics
The Johns Hopkins University School of Medicine
Baltimore, Maryland

Colleen McCormick MD
Department of Gynecology and Obstetrics
The Johns Hopkins University School of Medicine
Baltimore, Maryland

Wendy Monthly MD
Department of Gynecology and Obstetrics
The Johns Hopkins University School of Medicine
Baltimore, Maryland

Patricia Moore MD
Department of Gynecology and Obstetrics
The Johns Hopkins University School of Medicine
Baltimore, Maryland

Andrea Nugent MD
Department of Gynecology and Obstetrics
The Johns Hopkins University School of Medicine
Baltimore, Maryland

Courtney Rhoades MD
Department of Gynecology and Obstetrics
The Johns Hopkins University School of Medicine
Baltimore, Maryland

Francisco Rojas MD
Department of Gynecology and Obstetrics
The Johns Hopkins University School of Medicine
Baltimore, Maryland

Brenda Ross MD
Department of Gynecology and Obstetrics
The Johns Hopkins University School of Medicine
Baltimore, Maryland

Eli Rybak MD
Department of Gynecology and Obstetrics
The Johns Hopkins University School of Medicine
Baltimore, Maryland

Fiona Simpkins MD
Department of Gynecology and Obstetrics
The Johns Hopkins University School of Medicine
Baltimore, Maryland

Javier Soto MD
Department of Gynecology and Obstetrics
The Johns Hopkins University School of Medicine
Baltimore, Maryland

Lisa Soule MD
Department of Gynecology and Obstetrics
The Johns Hopkins University School of Medicine
Baltimore, Maryland

Muna Tahlak MD
Department of Gynecology and Obstetrics
The Johns Hopkins University School of Medicine
Baltimore, Maryland

Michelle Taylor MD
Department of Gynecology and Obstetrics
The Johns Hopkins University School of Medicine
Baltimore, Maryland

Dana Virgo MD
Department of Gynecology and Obstetrics
The Johns Hopkins University School of Medicine
Baltimore, Maryland

Nikos Vlahos MD
Department of Gynecology and Obstetrics
The Johns Hopkins University School of Medicine
Baltimore, Maryland

Edward Wallach MD
Department of Gynecology and Obstetrics
The Johns Hopkins University School of Medicine
Baltimore, Maryland

Shannon Walsh MD
Department of Gynecology and Obstetrics
The Johns Hopkins University School of Medicine
Baltimore, Maryland

Renée Ward MD
Department of Gynecology and Obstetrics
The Johns Hopkins University School of Medicine
Baltimore, Maryland

Frank Witter MD
Department of Gynecology and Obstetrics
The Johns Hopkins University School of Medicine
Baltimore, Maryland

Melissa Yates MD
Department of Gynecology and Obstetrics
The Johns Hopkins University School of Medicine
Baltimore, Maryland

Preface

A time-honored method for making the most of any learning experience is to be subjected to a test of knowledge acquired by that experience. Traditionally, this testing which begins in grade school and proceeds through college, graduate school and beyond, has been conducted in the confines of a classroom with the student undergoing quizzes, and final exams. This evaluation process forces that student to review and re-review the material covered by the examination. Even experienced physicians take state licensing board and national board exams as well as continuing certification under this model. Some CME tests cover material from lectures or reading material. However, the ubiquitous examination process is usually not very enjoyable. As physicians, we are fed our knowledge through various sources, but digest and synthesize it through daily clinical experiences. These experiences are truly exercises which make use of the factual and theoretical material which surround us in our day to day practice. As laborious as it is to prepare for and take exams, it is just as highly satisfying to experience the successful clinical application of our knowledge. This book is designed to be a fun-filled, clinically relevant learning experience based on factual material which has been translated to pertain to specific clinical situations and accompanied by a testing process.

The factual material is derived from the Johns Hopkins Manual of Gynecology and Obstetrics. This book was originally developed 6 years ago by the house staff and faculty of the Department of Gynecology and Obstetrics of the Johns Hopkins University School of Medicine and Johns Hopkins Hospital. Over 16,000 copies of the first two editions have sold worldwide and a 3rd edition is currently underway. This companion piece was the brain-child of Dr. Brandon Bankowski who has served as the Senior House Office editorial Board member of the manual. Each chapter corresponds to its respective chapter in the manual. The chapter consist of representative cases, as diverse as the practice of OB/GYN itself, which are immediately followed by test questions to challenge the reader and subsequently a series of feedback statements expressing the rationale for the correct answer.

This review is tailored to translate the material in the Manual into the language of your clinical mind. As with the Manual, this companion piece is the product of a joint effort by OB/GYN house staff, fellows, and faculty at Johns Hopkins. We hope that you enjoy this learning experience.

Edward E. Wallach, M.D.
J. Donald Woodruff Professor of Gynecology
Johns Hopkins Medical Institution
Department of Gynecology and Obstetrics

Primary and Preventive Care

Colleen McCormick

1 You are in clinic and notice that the next patient on your schedule is a 43-year-old woman coming for her annual exam. She has Down syndrome and has lived in a group home for several years. She has moderate aortic stenosis, but is otherwise fairly healthy. What vaccinations should she be offered?

A. Hepatitis B

B. Influenza

C. Pneumococcus

D. Hepatitis A

E. Tetanus toxoid

F. MMR

G. A, B, C, & E

H. C, E, & F

I. A, B, D, & E

G Vaccinations for adults are often overlooked but can provide significant benefits. Hepatitis B vaccination is now included in the general series of vaccinations for children, but is fairly new, so most adults have not received it. Patients who are intravenous drug users, are on dialysis, have liver or renal disease, are health care workers, have a history of other sexually transmitted diseases, or are residents or staff of institutions are candidates for vaccination. The vaccine is a series of three injections and conveys life-long immunity. Influenza vaccinations are created each year in anticipation of which strains will be prevalent, so they must be repeated each year. Patients who are residents of a long-term care facility have lowered immune systems, have renal or cardiac disease, are diabetic, or are health care workers are all candidates. Pneumococcal vaccinations are appropriate for any patient with a chronic disease (cardiac, pulmonary, diabetes, chronic liver disease), asplenic patients, and immunocompromised patients. Vaccination usually conveys life-long immunity, although revaccination may be necessary after 5 years. Hepatitis A is appropriate for international travelers, health care workers, food service workers, and illegal drug users. Tetanus toxoid needs to be administered as a booster once every 10 years. MMR immunity status should be checked in college students, international travelers, and pregnant women, and revaccination should be offered to those who are nonimmune.

2 A 57-year-old postmenopausal woman sees you for her primary care. She is in good health, does not smoke, and has no personal or family history of myocardial infarction (MI). As part of her health care maintenance you checked her cholesterol. What is the goal for her low-density lipoprotein (LDL) level?

A. <160

B. <130

C. <100

B Target LDL is defined by risk factors. Risk factors include age > 45 in men and > 55 in women, postmenopausal status, family history of MI at age < 55 in a male family member or < 65 in a female family member, smoking, diabetes, and HDL < 35. For one risk factor the goal is < 160. For two or more risk factors the goal is < 130. For patients with diabetes or a personal history of coronary artery disease the goal is < 100.

3 A 32-year-old woman with no significant family history of cancer comes in for her health maintenance visit. What cancer screening should be offered to her?

A. Breast
B. Ovary
C. Colon
D. Cervix
E. Thyroid
F. Lymphoma/leukemia
G. A & E
H. A & B
I. B & C
J. A & D

J Breast cancer recommendations remain somewhat controversial, but women ages 20–40 should have clinical breast exams every 2–3 years. Women > 40 years old should have yearly clinical breast exams. Yearly mammograms are recommended screening for women > 50 years old. Currently there is no consensus for frequency of mammograms between ages 40 and 50, with recommendations varying from every year to every other year, to not at all. This woman should be screened with a clinical breast exam.

Unfortunately, there is no good screening method for ovarian cancer. Likewise, there are no current recommendations for screening for thyroid cancer or leukemia/lymphoma.

There are several different sets of recommendations for colon cancer screening, including fecal occult blood screening every year, flexible sigmoidoscopy every 3–5 years, or colonoscopy every 5–10 years. All screening recommendations start at age 50.

All women who are sexually active or > 21 years old should be screened for cervical cancer with a Papanicolaou test. Yearly testing is recommended (although after three consecutive normal tests, women at low risk [not sexually active, no history of sexually transmitted diseases, in a mutually monogamous relationship] can be screened every 3 years instead).

2

Diseases of the Breast

Wendy Monthy

1 A 56-year-old postmenopausal woman presents to her gynecologist for a routine annual exam. While performing the breast examination, a 1-cm firm but nontender mass with indistinct borders is noted in her left breast.

The most appropriate imaging study upon detection of this mass is

A. Diagnostic mammography

B. Ultrasonography

C. Magnetic resonance imaging

D. Computed tomography

A When the presence of a lesion has already been detected, either as the result of physical examination or screening mammography, diagnostic mammography is used. Diagnostic mammography includes a more sophisticated approach such as spot compression views and magnification images. The mammogram is essential in evaluating other areas of the breast and the contralateral breast. Mammographic abnormalities suggestive of breast cancer include spiculated soft tissue densities, microcalcifications, and architectural distortion of the breast without obvious mass. Ultrasonography does not substitute for mammography. However, ultrasound is a common tool for distinguishing cystic from solid lesions. Magnetic resonance imaging (MRI) is beginning to play a more significant role in selected patients to evaluate the structure of and, when used with contrast, the blood flow in the lesion.

2 While the patient in Question 1 is in the office, the gynecologist decides to perform a fine-needle aspiration (FNA) of this solid breast mass, which yields a bloody aspirate. The next step in management should be to

A. Have the patient return in 4 weeks for a follow-up breast exam and repeat FNA if the lesion persists

B. Schedule the patient for lumpectomy with a general surgeon

C. Arrange for an excisional biopsy

D. Prescribe an antibiotic, as this is most likely due to an infection

C Fine-needle aspiration is traditionally used to obtain material from a breast abnormality for cytologic evaluation. It involves introduction of a narrow-gauge needle into the lesion. Although it is accurate in detecting malignant cells, it often cannot distinguish between invasive and noninvasive carcinomas. Any mass that does not disappear on aspiration, yields bloody aspirate, or does not completely resolve on ultrasound is an indication for core or excisional biopsy. Core biopsy, using a large-bore needle, reveals clinically more useful histologic information than FNA. Excisional biopsy, performed under local anesthesia, involves complete removal of the abnormality.

3 After pathologic examination, the patient in Question 1 is diagnosed with ductal carcinoma *in situ* (DCIS). Which of the following statements regarding this disease is *false*?

A. In DCIS, the risk for nodal involvement is about 40%, and therefore breast conservation therapy is not a treatment option.

B. With the increased use of mammography, showing diffuse microcalcifications, DCIS is being diagnosed with increased frequency.

C. DCIS can be divided into multiple histologic subtypes: solid, micropapillary, cribriform, and comedo.

D. DCIS refers to a proliferation of cancer cells within the ducts without invasion through the basement membrane into the surrounding stroma.

A Patients who have DCIS can be offered mastectomy or breast conservation therapy (BCT). In contrast to infiltrating cancer, the risk of nodal involvement is less than 1% in DCIS, so lymph node sampling is not recommended. The patient may elect mastectomy or undergo lumpectomy followed by radiation therapy. In some cases of multifocal disease, breast conservation therapy is contraindicated.

3

Critical Care

Alice Chung

1 A 38-year-old woman with past medical history significant for breast cancer is status post an uncomplicated total abdominal hysterectomy (TAH) and bilateral salpingophorectomy (BSO). On postoperative day 2, her vital signs are as follows: temperature 37.8°C, pulse 120, respiratory rate 18, blood pressure 110/60, and oxygen saturation 88% on room air. An arterial blood gas is drawn on room air, and her pH is 7.35, P_{O_2} is 58, P_{CO_2} is 35, and HCO_3 is 23. P_{IMAX} is 100 mm H_2O. Which of the following is the most likely etiology for her oxygen desaturation?

A. Opiate respiratory depression

B. Respiratory muscle weakness

C. Pulmonary embolism

D. Sepsis

C There are two types of respiratory failure, hypoxic and hypercapnic. Acute hypoxic respiratory failure occurs when the arterial P_{O_2} is less than 60 mm Hg or the arterial oxygen saturation is $< 90\%$, whereas hypercapnic respiratory failure occurs when the Pa_{CO_2} is > 46 mm Hg and pH is less than 7.35. It is helpful to calculate the A–a gradient in evaluating acute respiratory failure. The A–a gradient is increased in cardiopulmonary disorders (increased dead-space ventilation or intrapulmonary shunt) or a systemic oxygen delivery/uptake imbalance. In this patient, the A–a gradient is 48. (A–a gradient $= 148 - 1.2Pa_{CO_2} - P_{O_2}$) Her surgery and her past medical history of breast cancer are both risk factors for deep vein thrombosis and pulmonary embolism.

2 Which of the following is most effective in distinguishing cardiogenic and noncardiogenic pulmonary edema?

A. Central venous pressure

B. Pulmonary capillary wedge pressure

C. Cardiac index

D. Systemic vascular resistance index

B The Swan-Ganz catheter is placed in the subclavian or internal jugular vein. The tip of the catheter is guided through the right atrium, the right ventricle, and into the pulmonary artery. The pressure waveforms allow measurements of the pulmonary capillary wedge pressure (PCWP), which is a reflection of the left atrial pressure and the left diastolic ventricular pressure (as long as there is no obstruction between the left atrium and left ventricle). A normal PCWP is 6–12 mm Hg. In patients with cardiogenic pulmonary edema, the PCWP is elevated secondary to left ventricular systolic or diastolic dysfunction. In patients who have congestive heart failure and poor oxygenation or pulmonary infiltrates, the Swan-Ganz catheter is helpful in distinguishing between adult respiratory distress syndrome and cardiogenic pulmonary edema.

3 A 72-year-old woman is status post-BSO for an ovarian mass that has been discovered to be a mucinous cystadenoma. She has a history of diabetes mellitus controlled by oral hypoglycemic medications and 10 years of heavy tobacco use. On postoperative day 1, her urine output was 170 cc over 8 hours. Her weight is stable and her vital signs are within normal limits. A urinalysis, microscopy, urine electrolytes, and a basic metabolic panel are ordered. The specific gravity of her urine is 1.022. Urine microscopy is unremarkable. Urine creatinine is 112 mg/dL, urine sodium is 20 mEq/L. Her serum creatinine is 1.1 and her serum sodium is 140. What is the most likely cause of her oliguria?

A. Intravascular depletion

B. Acute tubular necrosis

C. Acute glomerulonephritis

D. Intraoperative ureter transection

A Oliguria is defined as urine output less than 400 cc per day. The causes of oliguria can be broken down to prerenal, renal, and postrenal disorders. In this patient her specific gravity was top normal and her fractional excretion (FE) of sodium was 0.7%.

$$\frac{(\text{Urine Na}/\text{plasma Na})}{(\text{Urine Cr}/\text{plasma Cr})} \times 100 = \text{FE}_{\text{Na}}$$

Urine microscopy is helpful in distinguishing intrinsic disorders by the presence of tubular epithelial cells and epithelial cell casts for acute tubular necrosis versus white cell casts for interstitial nephritis. If a postrenal disorder is suspected, placement of a Foley catheter and urinary tract ultrasonography are helpful.

4 A 78-year-old woman is status post an exploratory laparotomy, TAH-BSO, bilateral lymph node dissection, and tumor debulking for a stage IIIC serous ovarian carcinoma. On the night of surgery, the patient becomes tachypneic and is found in respiratory distress. An arterial blood gas on room air is as follows: pH 7.30, P_{CO_2} 60 mm Hg, Pa_{O_2} 53 mm Hg. She is transferred to the adult intensive care unit for intubation. What is the most appropriate mode of mechanical ventilation?

A. Assist-control ventilation

B. Intermittent mandatory ventilation

C. Pressure-controlled ventilation

D. Inverse-ratio ventilation

E. Pressure-support ventilation

B Mechanical ventilation should be considered in patients with respiratory distress. More specifically, if mechanical ventilation should be employed if the respiratory rate is greater than 35 breaths per minute, Pa_{O_2} is less than 60 mm Hg, Pa_{CO_2} is greater than 46 mm Hg with a pH less than 7.35, and absent gag reflex. Once the decision is made to intubate a patient, the mode of ventilation must be chosen. Pressure-controlled ventilation is appropriate for patients with neuromuscular disease. Inverse-ratio ventilation is indicated in patients with refractory hypoxemia or hypercapnia in patients with acute respiratory distress syndrome (ARDS) with conventional modes of ventilation. Assist-control ventilation delivers a breath at a preset controlled rate and volume when the patient cannot initiate a breath. When the patient breathes spontaneously, the ventilator assists each breath. In tachypneic patients, assist-control ventilation can lead to lung hyperinflation and respiratory alkalosis because it does not resolve their tachypnea. In contrast, intermittent mandatory ventilation delivers a breath at a preset rate and volume, but allows the patient to breathe at a spontaneous rate and volume between machine breaths without assistance. Synchronized intermittent mandatory ventilation prevents respiratory alkalosis and respiratory alkalosis by synchronizing spontaneous and machine respirations.

5 A 52-year-old woman is status post surgery and is noted to have deceased urine output. Urine osmoles are checked and they are 200 mOsm/L. Her serum sodium is 122 mEq/L. She weighs 70 kg. At what rate should she be repleted with 3% NaCl?

A. 26 cc per hour
B. 34 cc per hour
C. 41 cc per hour
D. 50 cc per hour

B Hyponatremia is defined as a serum sodium level less than 135 mEq/L. Hyponatremia is classified into three types by assessing extracellular volume: low, normal, and high. In patients with syndrome of inappropriate anti-diuretic hormone (ADH) (SIADH), the extracellular volume is normal and the urine osmolality is greater than 100, which has occurred in this patient. It is important to remember that sodium replacement must be repleted no greater than 0.5 mEq/L per hour. The goal is to replete the patient's sodium to 130 mEq/L. If the hyponatremia is corrected too quickly, central pontine myelinolyis can occur. In calculating the repletion of a patient's sodium, the total body water and sodium deficit are calculated.

The total body water (liters) is 50% of the lean body weight (kg) in women. The sodium deficit (mEq) is the normal total body water multiplied by (130 – current serum sodium level). The volume of 3% NaCl needed is calculated by the sodium deficit divided by 513 mEq/L, as each liter of 3% NaCl contains 513 mEq of sodium. Because it is important to replace the sodium no more rapidly than 0.5 mEq/L per hour, the number of hours for corrections is (130 – current sodium level) divided by 0.5. The fluid rate is then calculated by dividing the volume of hypertonic solution needed by the number of hours needed.

4

Preconception Counseling and Prenatal Care

Shannon Walsh

1 A 31-year-old gravida 0 presents to your office for a routine gynecologic exam, and reports that she and her husband are considering trying to conceive in the near future. The patient has an unremarkable medical, surgical, gynecologic, and family history. She and her husband are both of Northern European descent. She currently works in a day care center. In addition to routine preconceptual screening tests, you offer her:

A. Genetic carrier screening for hemoglobinopathies, Tay-Sachs disease, and Canavan's disease

B. Screening for parental karyotype

C. Cytomegalovirus and parvovirus B19 IgG screening

D. Tuberculosis testing

E. Hepatitis C screening

C Cytomegalovirus screening should be offered preconceptually to women who work in neonatal intensive care units, child care facilities, or dialysis units. Parvovirus B19 IgG screening may be offered to schoolteachers and child care workers. The patient's history does not support any of the other tests.

2 A 34-year-old gravida 1 para 1001 presents to your office reporting that she would like to try to conceive with her husband. She delivered her last child at term, and the child had a myelomeningocele. She is wondering what she can do to prevent a recurrence of this anomaly in a future pregnancy. You advise her to begin taking:

A. Prenatal vitamins once daily

B. 0.4 mg folate daily

C. 1.0 mg folate daily

D. 2.0 mg folate daily

E. 4.0 mg folate daily

E Couples with a prior child with a neural tube defect (NTD) have a recurrence risk of approximately 2%. Women who have previously carried a child with a NTD should take 4.0 mg of folic acid daily, unless contraindicated by the presence of pernicious anemia.

3 A 17-year-old gravida 2 para 0010 presents for her first prenatal visit at 11-3/7 weeks' gestation by unsure last menstrual period. In the course of the history, you learn that she smokes approximately 1 pack of cigarettes per day. You counsel her that cigarette smoking increases her risk of:

A. Fetal growth retardation, facial anomalies, and central nervous system (CNS) dysfunction

B. Spontaneous abortion, placenta previa, preterm rupture of membranes (PROM), low birthweight, and sudden infant death syndrome

C. Preterm delivery, fetal death *in utero*, cerebral infarction, microcephaly, and limb reduction deficits

D. Fetal visual and hearing deficits, including cataracts and glaucoma

E. Fetal hepatosplenomegaly, jaundice, and microcephaly with periventricular calcifications

B Smoking is associated with increased risk of spontaneous abortion (1.2–1.8 times greater in smokers), abortion of chromosomally normal fetus (39% more likely in smokers), abruptio placentae, placenta previa, PROM, preterm birth (1.2–1.5 times increased risk in smokers), low infant birthweight, and sudden infant death syndrome.

4 A 25-year-old marathon runner presents for her first prenatal visit at 7 weeks' gestation and inquires about whether she can continue her exercise regimen during the pregnancy. You advise her that:

A. She should stop running, as the impact could be harmful to the fetus.

B. She should consider switching to a weight-bearing form of exercise, as it may allow her to continue exercising comfortably throughout her pregnancy.

C. She should continue her exercise regimen without modification.

D. She should continue her exercise regimen, but modify the intensity of exercise in response to fatigue and shortness of breath, and ensure adequate nutrition and hydration.

D Continued exercise is very healthy in pregnancy, but women who engage in non-weight-bearing exercise are more likely to continue their exercise regimen throughout pregnancy. Pregnant women should not exercise to exhaustion, and should stop exercising if they begin to feel short of breath or extremely fatigued. Any exercise that poses a risk of abdominal trauma should be avoided. Pregnant women should be sure to maintain adequate hydration and wear appropriate clothing, and need to maintain an adequate diet. Women with pregnancy induced hypertension (PIH), preterm rupture of membranes (PROM), history of preterm labor or incompetent cervix, persistent second- or third-trimester bleeding, or intrauterine growth retardation (IUGR) should avoid exercise during pregnancy.

5 A 43-year-old gravid woman presents to you with concerns about her child's risk for chromosomal abnormalities. In addition to referring her for prenatal genetic counseling, you may recommend:

A. First-trimester hCG and PAPP-A levels, in addition to nuchal translucency measurement at 10–14 weeks.

B. Triple-screen testing and complete anomaly ultrasound
C. Chorionic villus sampling (CVS) testing
D. Amniocentesis
E. All of the above

E All of the above options are appropriate tests to recommend, and which is/are right for each patient depends on the individual patient, her wishes regarding invasive versus noninvasive testing, and her plans for continuing or terminating the pregnancy should the test results be abnormal. First-trimester screening is thought to detect approximately 85–90% of Down syndrome, but it is unclear how well it detects other abnormalities, including trisomy 18. Triple-screen testing can detect increased probability of Down syndrome, NTDs, and trisomy 18. Amniocentesis and CVS testing can more definitively diagnose chromosomal abnormalities, but there is a risk of cytogenetically ambiguous results secondary to maternal cell contamination or mosaicism. Amniocentesis can also more definitively diagnose NTDs.

5

Normal Labor and Delivery, Operative Delivery, and Malpresentations

Amy Hearne

Please read the following vignette to answer Questions 1–3.
A 24-year-old gravida 2 para 1001 at 39-5/7 weeks' gestation was admitted to the labor and delivery suite in active labor at 5 cm dilation, 50% effaced, and −1 station. She received an epidural and progressed to full dilation. She pushed for 50 minutes to deliver a vigorous female infant. The placenta was then delivered 40 minutes later.

---

1 Which of the following statements is false?

A. The patient had a prolonged second stage of labor.

B. The patient had a prolonged third stage of labor.

C. The 5th-percentile of rate of maximal dilation for this patient is 1.5 cm per hour.

B The second stage of labor is the interval between full dilation and delivery of the infant. The average duration is 50 minutes for nulliparas and 20 minutes for multiparas. The second stage is considered prolonged after 2 hours in nulliparous patients and 1 hour in multiparous patients, with an additional hour allowed if the patient has received epidural anesthesia. This patient's second stage of labor was 50 minutes, which is not prolonged. The third stage of labor is the interval between delivery of the infant and delivery of the placenta, umbilical cord, and fetal membranes. The average is 10 minutes and it is considered prolonged if it lasts greater than 30 minutes. The 5th percentile for maximal dilation is 1.5 cm per hour for multiparous and 1.2 cm per hour for nulliparous patients.

2 The correct order of the seven cardinal movements of labor for this patient should be

A. Engagement, descent, flexion, internal rotation, extension, external rotation, expulsion

B. Flexion, descent, engagement, internal rotation, extension, external rotation, expulsion

C. Descent, engagement, flexion, internal rotation, extension, external rotation, expulsion

D. Engagement, descent, flexion, internal rotation, external rotation, extension, expulsion

A The seven cardinal movements of labor refer to changes in position of the fetal head during passage through the birth canal. The following is the correct order: engagement, descent, flexion, internal rotation, extension, external rotation.

3 What is this patient's pelvis type if her pelvic inlet is rounded, side walls are straight, and the sacrum is well curved?

A. Anthropoid

B. Android

C. Platypelloid

D. Gynecoid

D This patient's pelvis type is gynecoid. This type of pelvis is found in 40–50% of women. In a patient with an anthropoid pelvis the inlet is oval, long, and narrow; the side walls are straight; the sacrum is long and narrow; and the sacrosciatic notch is wide. In a patient with an android pelvis, the inlet is heart-shaped with a short posterior sagittal diameter. In a patient with a platypelloid pelvis, the inlet is flat and oval with a short posterior diameter.

Please read the following vignette to answer Questions 4 and 5.

A 28-year-old gravida 3 para 2002 at 39-5/7 weeks' gestation presents to the labor and delivery suite in active labor. Her obstetric history is significant for two full-term spontaneous vaginal deliveries with infants weighing 3,840 and 3,750 g. During this pregnancy the patient has been diagnosed with Class A2 gestational diabetes. At delivery a shoulder dystocia is encountered.

---

4 Which of the following is not a risk factor for shoulder dystocia?

A. Maternal obesity

B. Estimated fetal weight of 4,000 g

C. Gestational diabetes

D. Hypertension

E. Previous macrosomic infant

D Risk factors associated with shoulder dystocia are fetal macrosomia, history of macrosomic infant, maternal obesity, diabetes, and post-term pregnancy. Hypertension is not associated with shoulder dystocia.

5 Which of the following should you not do if you encounter a shoulder dystocia?

A. Call for help and check the clock

B. McRoberts maneuver

C. Fundal pressure

D. Suprapubic pressure

E. Episiotomy

C Fundal pressure should *not* be applied, as it presses the fetal shoulder into the pubic symphysis and may lead to uterine rupture. If a shoulder dystocia is encountered, the health care provider should call for help, note the time, perform an episiotomy, perform a McRoberts maneuver, and have an assistant apply suprapubic pressure. If those maneuvers are not successful, consider second-line maneuvers such as the wood corkscrew, clavicle fracture, symphysiotomy, or Zavanelli maneuver.

Please read the following vignette to answer Questions 6–8. A 30-year-old gravida 2 para 0101 at 36 weeks' gestation presents for routine prenatal care. On Leopold's maneuver the fetus is found to be in the breech presentation.

---

6 Leopold's maneuvers are a series of abdominal palpations of the gravid uterus to ascertain both fetal lie and presentation.

A. True

B. False

A **True.** Leopold's maneuvers are a series of palpations of the gravid uterus to ascertain fetal lie and presentation. The fundus is palpated to ascertain the presence or absence and nature of the fetal pole. The lateral walls of the uterus are examined. The nature and station of the presenting part is determined by palpating above the pubic symphysis.

7 Which of the following statements is false?

A. Breech presentation occurs in approximately 25% of pregnancies at 28 weeks' gestation, 7% of pregnancies at 32 weeks' gestation, and 3–4% of term pregnancies in labor.

B. Complete breech occurs when the fetus has one or both hips extended.

C. Frank breech occurs when the fetus is flexed at both hips and extended at both knees.

D. Breech presentation is associated with risk of cord prolapse.

E. External cephalic version can be offered to most patients with a breech fetus at term.

B Complete breech occurs when the fetus is flexed at the hips and flexed at the knees. Incomplete or footling breech occurs when the fetus has one or both hips extended. Frank breech occurs when the fetus has both hips flexed and both knees extended. The incidence of the breech presentation is approximately 25% at less than 28 weeks' gestation, 7% at 32 weeks' gestation, and 3–4% at term. The risks associated with breech presentation include cord prolapse. External cephalic version (ECV) can be offered to most patients with a breech fetus at term. Contraindications to ECV include third-trimester bleeding, oligohydramnios, ruptured membranes, and any other contraindication to labor or vaginal delivery (placenta previa, prior classical cesarean section, etc.).

8 The Mauriceau-Smellie-Veit maneuver places downward traction on the mandible.

A. True

B. False

B **False.** During breech delivery the infant's head should be delivered in the flexed position. If the neck is hyperextended, the risk of spinal cord injury increases. The Mauriceau-Smellie-Veit maneuver places downward traction on the maxilla. Do not apply pressure on the mandible, as it can cause dislocation or subluxation of the mandible.

Please read the following vignette to answer Questions 9 and 10.

A 32-year-old nullipara presents for induction of labor at 41-2/7 weeks' gestation. Her cervical exam at admission was 1 cm dilated, 50% effaced, −2 station, medium consistency, posterior position. She received prostaglandins for cervical ripening. She eventually progressed to full dilation and pushed until +3 station with epidural anesthesia. The patient was then delivered with forceps due to a nonreassuring fetal heart tracing.

---

9 The patient's Bishop score was

A. 3

B. 4

C. 5

D. 6

B The Bishop score for this patient was 4. The Bishop score is a way of assessing the state of the cervix at the time of induction and can be related to the success of labor induction.

10 Which of the following is true?

A. Prepidil gel is injected intravaginally.

B. Cervadil is a vaginal insert containing 10 mg dinoprostone, which releases medication at a rate of 0.3 mg per hour.

C. Cytotec (25 μg) can be inserted intravaginally every 3–4 hours.

D. A Bishop score of more than 8 requires cervical ripening.

B Prepidil is a prostaglandin E2 gel that contains 0.5 mg of dinoprostone in a 2.5-mL syringe that is injected intracervically up to every 6 hours, up to three doses in 24 hours. Cervadil (prostaglandin E2) is a vaginal insert containing 10 mg of dinoprostone that releases medication at a rate of 0.3 mg per hour. Cytotec is a prostaglandin E1, not a prostaglandin E2. When the Bishop score is more than 8, the likelihood of vaginal delivery after induction of labor is similar to that with spontaneous labor.

11 This patient had an outlet forceps delivery.

A. True

B. False

B **False.** This patient had a low forceps-assisted vaginal delivery. The type of forceps delivery is classified by station. With outlet forceps the scalp is visible without separating the labia, the skull has reached the pelvic floor, the head is at or on the perineum, and the head is either direct anterior-posterior or does not require more than 45 degrees of rotation to accomplish this. With low forceps the station is +2 or greater. With mid forceps the head is engaged but above +2 station.

6

Fetal Assessment

Dana Gossett
Karin Blakemore

1 Your patient is a 27-year-old gravida 2 para 1001 at 22 weeks' gestation with a history of chronic hypertension. She has some evidence of chronic renal insufficiency based on microalbuminuria. During this pregnancy, she has been taking Aldomet to control her blood pressures with good results. Her last pregnancy was complicated by superimposed preeclampsia and HELLP syndrome, necessitating delivery at 33 weeks. She is concerned about the prognosis for this pregnancy, and asks you what you are going to do to check on her baby. You recommend:

A. Weekly nonstress tests (NSTs) starting at this visit

B. Weekly NSTs or biophysical profile (BPP) starting at 28 weeks' gestation

C. Weekly NSTs starting at 36 weeks' gestation

D. Weekly Doppler flow alone starting at 28 weeks' gestation

E. No testing unless her blood pressure rises to 140/90

B An NST is not appropriate prior to the age of viability (24 weeks' gestation), nor are there standards for its interpretation. B would certainly be a reasonable option for testing. Because many fetuses do not routinely demonstrate reactivity on their NSTs before 32 weeks' gestation, you may need to do further testing, e.g., a biophysical profile. In general, when there is a past history of poor pregnancy outcome, you should initiate testing prior to the gestational age at which that outcome occurred, in this case prior to 33 weeks. At the present time there is very little evidence to support the use of Doppler ultrasound as the sole means of fetal testing. While it can provide a useful adjunct to other evaluations of fetal well-being, there is insufficient evidence at present to use Doppler alone. Given the association between chronic hypertension and placental insufficiency, testing is warranted during the third trimester.

2 A patient who is not registered for prenatal care comes to the labor and delivery suite complaining of decreased fetal movement for the last 2 days. She denies any medical problems, but says that she hasn't been feeling well this week, and hasn't been eating much. She tells you her due date, which she says is based on a first-trimester sonogram done in the emergency room. You confirm that this sonogram exists, and you calculate that she is at 35 weeks' gestation. She is placed on a fetal cardiotocometer and uterine tocodynomometer. The fetal heart rate is in the 150s with average short- and long-term variability, and is nonreactive after 30 minutes. Which of the following would *not* explain the nonreactive tracing?

A. Fetal sleep cycle
B. Maternal smoking
C. Maternal substance abuse
D. Gestational age
E. Poor maternal oral intake

D Fetal sleep cycles can last up to 80 minutes. Therefore, one option for management would be to monitor the fetus longer. If the patient has smoked recently, this may result in a transiently nonreactive tracing. However, further monitoring until the fetus is reactive, or additional antenatal testing, must be performed to ensure fetal well-being. Certainly, the use of opiates and sedatives as well as other legal drugs such as beta-blockers, can explain a nonreactive fetal tracing. A medication and drug history as well as a toxicology screen would be appropriate. Again, however, further investigation must be done to ensure fetal well-being. Nonstress tests should routinely be reactive after

32 weeks' gestation. Beyond 32 weeks's gestation, a nonreactive nonstress test should be considered abnormal. If the patient has not eaten in several days, then hypoglycemia may be the explanation for poor fetal testing. Intravenous hydration with a dextrose solution should be considered. Oral rehydration should be considered very carefully; if the fetal status should deteriorate during your evaluation, urgent delivery may become necessary, and her anesthetic risk will be lower if she has remained NPO.

7

Complications of Labor and Delivery

Shari Lawson

Please read the following vignette to answer Questions 1–3. A 27-year-old gravida 6 para 5015 has developed a postpartum hemorrhage following a spontaneous vaginal delivery. She was admitted 2 days ago for induction of labor and received 36 hours of oxytocin prior to delivery.

---

1 The most common cause of postpartum hemorrhage is

A. Uterine atony
B. Cervical, vaginal, or perineal lacerations
C. Retained products of conception
D. Coagulopathy

A The most common cause of postpartum hemorrhage is uterine atony. Uterine contraction following delivery constricts the spiral arterioles in the myometrium and controls bleeding. Predisposing factors to postpartum hemorrhage include grand multiparity, uterine distension due to multifetal gestation or polyhydramnios, prolonged administration of oxytocin, and chorioamnionitis.

2 Following bimanual massage, a uterine contractile agent is administered. Which of the agents listed below is contraindicated in a patient with chronic hypertension or preeclampsia?

A. Oxytocin

B. Methylergonovine maleate

C. 15-Methylprostaglandin $F_{2\alpha}$

D. Dinoprostin

E. Misoprostol

B Methylergonovine maleate (Methergine), a potent vasoconstrictor, is contraindicated in a patient with chronic hypertension or preeclampsia. 15-Methylprostaglandin (Hemabate) and dinoprostin are relatively contraindicated in an asthmatic patient.

Please read the following vignette to answer Questions 4 and 5.

A 16-year-old gravida 1 para 0 at 39 weeks' gestation estimated gestational age presents to labor and delivery following premature rupture of membranes. Her cervix is 2 cm dilated. After 6 hours, her cervical exam is unchanged and oxytocin induction is initiated. Epidural anesthesia is administered. The patient's progress in labor is slow and an intrauterine pressure catheter is placed to assess the strength of her contractions. She has several sterile vaginal exams performed. Twenty-four hours after rupture of membranes, the patient has not yet delivered and has developed a temperature of 38.0°C (100.4°F).

---

3 The most likely etiology for the fever is

A. Epidural fever

B. Chorioamnionitis

C. Drug reaction to oxytocin

D. Aspiration pneumonia

B This patient's fever is likely due to chorioamnionitis. She has several predisposing risk factors, including prolonged rupture of membranes, multiple vaginal exams, and internal monitoring. Other risk factors include low socioeconomic status, history of sexually transmitted infections, and preterm rupture of membranes.

4 Which of the following statements is true?

I. Chorioamnionitis should be treated with cefoxitin (or another second-generation cephalosporin) and doxycycline.

II. Chorioamnionitis is a polymicrobial infection.

III. Chorioamnionitis should be treated with ampicillin and gentamicin (or if the patient is penicillin-allergic, gentamicin and clindamycin).

IV. Chorioamnionitis is always diagnosed by Gram stain and bacterial culture of the amniotic fluid.

A. I only
B. II only
C. III only
D. IV only
E. I and II
F. II and III

F Chorioamnionitis is a polymicrobial infection. The diagnosis is usually made following clinical assessment of the patient. The following signs and symptoms are associated with chorioamnionitis: fever, maternal tachycardia, fetal tachycardia, fundal tenderness, leukocytosis, and foul-smelling vaginal discharge. It should be treated by delivery of the infant and antibiotic coverage using ampicillin and gentamicin in labor. Clindamycin may be substituted for ampicillin in the penicillin-allergic patient.

5 When seen in the infant, chest retractions, cyanosis, tachypnea, and coarse breath sounds may be an indicator of any of the following *except*

A. Amniotic fluid embolism
B. Transient tachypnea of the newborn
C. Meconium aspiration syndrome

A Both transient tachypnea of the newborn and meconium aspiration syndrome can cause respiratory distress in the newborn. Amniotic fluid embolism is rare and is a maternal complication resulting in clinical findings akin to anaphylactic shock in the mother.

Please read the following vignette to answer Question 6.
A 32-year-old gravida 1 para 1 presents to your office for a postpartum checkup. The patient reports that she has had foul-smelling yellowish-brown vaginal discharge since delivery. The patient's intrapartum course was complicated by a protracted first stage of labor lasting 36 hours. The second stage lasted 2.5 hours and necessitated a low forceps delivery for terminal bradycardia. The patient had a midline episiotomy performed that extended and completely transected the anal sphincter. The laceration was repaired in the labor and delivery room. On your exam, you note a fistulous tract between the posterior vagina and the rectum.

6 Rectovaginal fistulas occur when obstructed and prolonged labor causes pressure necrosis of the posterior vagina and rectovaginal septum.

A. True

B. False

B **False.** Rectovaginal fistulae are usually the result of obstetrical trauma (i.e., following instrument-assisted vaginal deliveries). Rectal examinations should be performed following any vaginal delivery during which rectal injury is suspected, so that any existing injury can be identified and repaired. Vesicovaginal fistulae occur when obstructed and prolonged labor causes pressure necrosis of the anterior vagina and vesicovaginal septum.

8

Gestational Complications

Dana Gossett
Edith Gurewitsch

1 A 25-year-old woman, gravida 1 para 0, presents to your office for her first prenatal visit at 10 weeks' gestation by a certain last menstrual period. On your pelvic exam, her uterus is equivalent to a 14 weeks' gestation. Sonography confirms a twin gestation, and a sac separation is seen between the two fetuses. The patient asks you what she should do differently now that she knows she is carrying twins. You advise all of the following *except*:

A. She will need to increase her caloric intake an additional 300 kcal per day.

B. She will need routine sonograms every 2–3 weeks starting at 23 weeks to evaluate fetal growth.

C. She is at higher risk for preterm delivery, and should remain on bedrest starting at 20 weeks' gestation.

D. She is likely to need a cesarean section for delivery.

E. Her pregnancy may be at risk for twin–twin transfusion syndrome (TTTS).

C It is true that each additional fetus increases maternal caloric needs by 300 kcal per day. Sonograms for assessment of fetal growth should not be performed more frequently than every 3–4 weeks, as the margin of error on the sonographic measurements may be greater than the potential growth for shorter intervals. There is little evidence to support routine prescription of bedrest in uncomplicated twin pregnancies. Bedrest can have both psychological effects and medical complications (e.g., venous thrombosis), and should therefore not be considered a benign intervention.

More than 80% of twin gestations will have a vertex presentation of twin A, and therefore be potentially eligible for vaginal delivery. The patient can be advised that cesarean section rates are higher for twin gestations than for singletons, but that decisions regarding her delivery will be based on the positions of the fetuses as well as other clinical factors. A sac separation was visualized between the two fetuses on sonogram. This means that the gestation is either dichorionic/diamniotic or monochorionic/diamniotic. Until placentation is definitively established by seeing or not seeing a "twin peak sign" (implying dichorionicity), her risk for TTTS cannot be established. TTTS occurs most commonly with monochorionic/diamniotic gestation, but even in this setting it is quite rare.

2 One of your obstetric patients presents for her office visit at 32 weeks' gestation. She is feeling well and has no concerns. On exam, her fundal height is 36 cm. You review your records, and see that at 28 weeks' gestation her fundal height was 30 cm; at 24 weeks it was 25 cm. The patient's weight is 295 lb; she has gained 38 lb since the beginning of the pregnancy. All of her laboratory studies have been normal. Your next step is

A. Continue routine prenatal care, which in your office means seeing the patient again in 2 weeks.

B. Bring the patient back in 1 week for another measurement and a nutrition consult. Her fundal height is most likely due to maternal obesity and excessive weight gain.

C. Obtain an ultrasound to assess fetal growth. She is at risk for a large infant because of her obesity and her excessive weight gain.

D. Repeat her glucose screen. She probably has a large baby because of undiagnosed gestational diabetes.

C When the fundal height and gestational age differ by more than 2, further investigation should be performed to determine the cause. Maternal obesity certainly may explain the excessive fundal height. However, one cannot assume this without an ultrasound. If a sonogram demonstrates a normally grown fetus and a normal amniotic fluid volume, only then can one assume that the large fundal height is due to the dimensions of the maternal abdomen. Sonography should be your next step. Not only will it evaluate the growth of the fetus, it can also diagnose polyhydramnios as a cause for size greater than dates. Without an ultrasound, you do not yet know that she has a large baby. Your measurements may simply reflect her abdominal fat stores. The first step should be an ultrasound.

3 For the patient described in Question 2, you choose to obtain a sonogram. Her last sonogram was at 21 weeks' gestation, at which time the fetal size was consistent with gestational age based on her last menstrual period. At this second sonogram, the fetal weight is at the 69th percentile, demonstrating normal growth, but the amniotic fluid index is 29 cm, giving her a diagnosis of polyhydramnios. You explain to the patient that:

A. You will need to repeat her glucose screen, to make sure she has not developed gestational diabetes since her 28 weeks' visit.

B. She is at increased risk for preterm delivery because of her polyhydramnios, and she should consider a therapeutic amniocentesis to reduce this risk.

C. Polyhydramnios is frequently associated with chromosomal anomalies and congenital infections, and she should consider a diagnostic amniocentesis for chromosomes and infectious serologies.

D. Her fetus is at increased risk for poor outcomes, and you recommend starting antenatal testing with nonstress tests.

A One of the most common reasons for isolated polyhydramnios is maternal diabetes. Although the patient had a normal glucose screen at 28 weeks' gestation, it would be wise to repeat the test in light of the increased fluid. In an asymptomatic patient with mild polyhydramnios, there is no indication for therapeutic amniocentesis. This procedure should be reserved for patients with severe polyhydramnios that is causing significant discomfort or dyspnea. Mild polyhydramnios is rarely associated with chromosomal or infectious causes. In severe cases, however, the rates of aneuploidy may be much higher. Unlike oligohydramnios, mild isolated polyhydramnios does not warrant antenatal surveillance.

4 Your obstetric patient presents to your office for a routine 36 weeks' visit complaining of decreased fetal movement. Fetal heart tones are auscultated in the 140s. Her fundal height is 32 cm. You do a quick ultrasound in your office, and find that she has an amniotic fluid index (AFI) of 3.2 cm. The fetal weight is at the 18th percentile. Your further evaluation should include all of the following *except*:

A. Pelvic examination to rule out rupture of membranes as a cause of the oligohydramnios

B. A nonstress test to evaluate her complaint of decreased fetal movement

C. Amniocentesis to assess fetal lung maturity

D. Aggressive IV hydration and repeat AFI in 2 hours

D Rupture of membranes should always be considered when oligohydramnios is diagnosed, not only in the term and near-term patient, but at any gestational age. Maternal perception of decreased fetal movement may simply be due to the low amniotic fluid volume. However, surveillance with a nonstress test should be performed. Oligohydramnios is not an indication for amniocentesis at this gestational age. In the term and near-term fetus, oligohydramnios is best managed by prompt delivery, and assessment of fetal lung maturity is not required. While maternal dehydration may lower amniotic fluid volume, there is no history in this patient to suggest this as the cause for her oligohydramnios. Additionally, it is unlikely that the AFI would change significantly over a 2-hour period.

5 Your patient is a 34-year-old gravida 3 para 2002 at 22 weeks' gestation. She presents to your office concerned about the findings on her recent sonogram. This sonogram, performed for routine anatomic evaluation, found that her fetus was lagging in growth by 2 weeks behind the expected size based on her certain last menstrual period (which was confirmed by an early ultrasound examination). The fetal measurements were symmetric (all were lagging equally), and the amniotic fluid volume was borderline low. There were no structural anomalies of the fetus or placenta noted. She asks you to explain the implications of these findings. You tell her:

A. Her dates are most likely wrong, and you are going to change her due date based on the ultrasound. She is really only 19 weeks pregnant.

B. Because all of the measurements are lagging equally, the fetus is most likely constitutionally small. She should have another ultrasound in 4 weeks to make sure that it is continuing to grow along its own growth curve.

C. Her fetus has intrauterine growth restriction (IUGR), probably due to placental insufficiency. She should remain at bedrest, optimize her nutritional intake and hydration, and stop any potentially harmful habits such as smoking or drinking alcohol.

D. Her fetus has intrauterine growth restriction (IUGR), and she needs an amniocentesis to determine the cause.

D If the patient is certain of her last menstrual period, her due date should not be changed based on a mid-trimester ultrasound. Instead, the finding of growth restriction should prompt further evaluation. It is not possible to distinguish between the constitutionally small fetus and the fetus with symmetric growth restriction on ultrasound. In either case, she will need further sonograms to assess growth. The fetal measurements are all lagging equally, rendering a diagnosis of symmetric IUGR. Symmetric IUGR is less likely than asymmetric IUGR to be caused by uteroplacental insufficiency, unless the uteroplacental insufficiency begins very early. Optimal nutrition and smoking cessation are important for any pregnancy, but are unlikely to reverse mid-trimester IUGR, except in the cases of severe malnutrition or very heavy maternal smoking. Because this fetus has mid-trimester, symmetric IUGR, as well as borderline oligohydramnios, both chromosomal and infectious etiologies need to be ruled out. Amniocentesis for karyotype and for infectious studies should be offered.

9

Preterm Labor and Premature Rupture of Membranes

Andrea Nugent
Jude Crino

1 A 24-year-old female gravida 3 para 2 at 28 weeks' gestation presents to Labor and Delivery complaining of contractions for the last 12 hours with a clear discharge. She appears flushed and in pain. Her pulse is 110 beats per minute, temperature 38.5°C, and blood pressure 92/57 mm Hg. On physical examination, she demonstrates tenderness over her uterine fundus. She has no costovertebral angle (CVA) tenderness. Her pelvic exam reveals muco-purulent discharge which turns the nitrazine paper bright blue. On microscopic exam there are many white blood cells (WBCs) with characteristic "ferning." Her cervix is closed. The fetal heartbeat has average to poor variability and the baseline remains in the 170s. She is contracting every 4 minutes. Her WBC count is elevated and her urine analysis shows many WBCs without bacteria. The most likely diagnosis is

A. Pyelonephritis

B. Pelvic inflammatory disease (PID)

C. Chorioamnionitis

D. Preterm labor

C The most likely diagnosis is chorioamnionitis. She demonstrates 3 signs and symptoms of this condition:

fundal tenderness, fetal, and maternal tachycardia. This is in association with premature rupture of membranes and frank pus coming from the cervical os. Although pyelonephritis is in the differential, she has no CVA tenderness or bacteruria; therefore, pyelonephritis is less likely. PID is highly unlikely at a gestational age of 28 weeks. PID is classically an ascending infection from the cervix into the uterus, fallopian tubes, and peritoneal cavity. Once a pregnancy fills the uterine cavity, this precludes the classic ascending infection (usually by 10–12 weeks' gestation). Although the patient is probably going into preterm labor due to infection, her cervix is closed and it is more likely that this started out as an infection, not preterm labor.

2 A 30-year-old gravida 1 para 0 at 30 weeks' gestation presents to Labor and Delivery complaining of "cramping" for the last 2–3 days. She has had no vaginal bleeding or leakage of fluid. The fetal movements are unchanged. She has no dysuria or hematuria. Placed on the monitor, she is found to be contracting irregularly every 6–7 minutes. Which test is the most predictive that she will not deliver within the next 2 weeks?

A. Sonographic cervical length of > 3 cm

B. A negative saline wet preparation for clue cells

C. A negative urine culture

D. A negative fetal fibronectin

E. A closed cervix on bimanual exam

D The absence of fetal fibronectin in cervical secretions has a 94% negative predictive value for preterm delivery. This means that a woman with a negative fetal fibronectin test has a 94% probability that she will not deliver within the next 2–3 weeks. On the other hand, its positive predictive value is much lower, and therefore, it cannot be used to diagnose preterm labor by itself. This test is limited to a gestational age of 24–36 weeks and cannot be used in patients who have demonstrated rupture of membranes or undergone recent cervical exam or sexual intercourse within the last 24 hours. It can be helpful in distinguishing between preterm labor and preterm contractions. In this way, one may avoid unnecessary tocolysis and the associated risks.

3 You have admitted a patient for preterm labor with demonstrated cervical change from closed last week in clinic to 3 cm of dilation. Upon taking her history, you find she is a 36-year-old gravida 1 para 0 who is at 27 weeks' gestation. She also has a significant past medical history of progressive weakness. She notices that her eyelids tend to tire and become almost closed after only a few hours of waking. She has recently seen a neurologist who has not gotten back to her with the results of her tests. Which tocolytic should be avoided as treatment for this patient's preterm labor?

A. Nifedipine

B. Indomethacin

C. Magnesium sulfate

D. Terbutaline

E. Ethanol

C Although the patient in question does not carry the diagnosis of myasthenia gravis, she has many of the signs and symptoms associated with the disease. Until it is clear that she does not have the disease, magnesium sulfate should be avoided because administration may cause acute cardiac toxicity in a patient with myasthenia gravis. Indomethacin would be a good choice for tocolysis, as she is less than 32 weeks' gestation. Nifedipine is not contraindicated in myasthenia gravis and neither is terbutaline.

4 A 19-year-old gravida 2 para 1 presents at 23 weeks' and 5 days' of gestation by a certain last menstrual period and a first-trimester ultrasound with preterm labor. Her cervical exam is 4 cm dilated and she is contracting every 2–3 minutes. She is immediately started on intravenous magnesium sulfate and given the appropriate corticosteroids. Her wet-preparation slide revealed clue cells, the KOH demonstrated a positive "whiff test," and the pH was >4.5. You decide to give her antibiotics. The best regimen would be

A. Ampicillin and gentamicin

B. Ciprofloxacin and metronidazole

C. Penicillin and metronidazole

D. Metronidazole

C When considering antibiotics for this patient one must consider two issues. First, she is very preterm and in active labor with an unknown group B streptococcal (GBS) status. Severely preterm infants are very susceptible to GBS infections and should have GBS prophylaxis during labor, even when GBS status is unknown. Therefore, one should administer penicillin to avoid the devastating consequences of preterm neonatal GBS sepsis. The other issue is that she has been diagnosed with bacterial vaginosis, which has been implicated as a potential cause of preterm labor and should be treated with metronidazole upon diagnosis. Ciprofloxacin is contraindicated in pregnancy, and ampicillin and gentamicin fail to cover the organisms in question.

5 You are called emergently to the Labor and Delivery suite for a patient who is on the stretcher writhing in pain, holding her abdomen. She is an 18-year-old gravida 2 para 1 at approximately 34 weeks' gestation without any prenatal care who started having pain of acute onset 1 hour earlier. She is contracting every 2 minutes. As you are taking her history, she proceeds to vomit and simultaneously, approximately 500 cc of blood is expelled from her vagina. Bedside ultrasonography reveals a 32-week fetus in a complete breech presentation with a heartbeat in the 160s, and an anterior placenta. A sterile speculum examination reveals a 2-cm-dilated cervix with 50% effacement. There is a steady stream of bright red blood coming from the cervical os. Your next immediate step is

A. Administer a 6-g bolus of intravenous magnesium sulfate, followed by 4 g per hour.

B. Immediate corticosteroid administration, followed by a subcutaneous injection of 0.25 mg of terbutaline.

C. Bedside emergency cesarean section.

D. Arrange for 2 units of cross-matched red blood cells.

E. Give 4 mg of morphine intravenously for pain.

D This patient is most likely experiencing abruptio placenta, or premature detachment of the implanted placenta from the uterine wall, the etiologies of which are outlined in Chapter 10. The important thing to note is that she is actively bleeding and runs the risk of disseminated intravascular coagulopathy, which may cause even more blood loss. Therefore, the next immediate step should be to arrange for 2 units of cross-matched red blood cells. Tocolytics would be contraindicated in this scenario until the maternal hemodynamic status has been assessed. One may consider tocolytics for the preterm gestation if both the mother and baby are hemodynamically stable. A bedside crash cesarean section is not necessary, as the fetal status is stable. Because of the breech fetal presentation and the likely uncontrolled bleeding, a controlled cesarean section may be warranted in the future; however, it would be prudent to arrange for blood and blood products prior to starting the procedure. Although pain control is important, delivery may be imminent and narcotics should be avoided to prevent neonatal respiratory depression. Narcotic use at this time may also mask symptoms of hypovolemic shock.

10

Third-Trimester Bleeding

Fiona Simpkins
Abimbola Aina

1 A 36-year-old gravida 2, para 1001 at 31 weeks' gestation with a history of painless vaginal bleeding presents to Labor and Delivery reporting another episode of vaginal bleeding. She has had chronic hypertension for 3 years and currently is taking 2 g/day α-methyldopa. She brings a blood-soaked towel with her, but she is not currently bleeding. She reports fetal movement, no loss of fluid, and no uterine contractions. Her blood pressure is 130/80 mm Hg, pulse 85 beats per minute. The fetal heart tracing shows a reassuring fetal heart rate. Ultrasound performed at the bedside reveals normal amniotic fluid volume, normal anterior placenta, and biometry appropriate for gestational age. A speculum examination reveals a slightly friable cervix, which appears long and closed. There is no pooling and no active bleeding. Her hemoglobin is 10.2 g/dL. Of the following options, the most likely diagnosis is

A. Cervical abrasion

B. Vasa previa

C. Succenturiate placental lobe

D. Placental abruption

E. Premature rupture of membranes

D Placental abruption (PA) is the premature separation of a normally implanted placenta. Its incidence is 1 per 250 deliveries. PA is associated with maternal hypertension, advanced maternal age, multiparity, cocaine use, tobacco use, chorioamnioitis, and trauma. PA may present dramatically with a nonreassuring fetal heart rate tracing or fetal demise and maternal hemorrhage, shock, and disseminated intravascular coagulation. Patients with placental abruption are often diagnosed retrospectively after delivery. Although the classic presentation is vaginal bleeding, abdominal pain, and an abnormal fetal heart rate tracing, the presenting problem is often idiopathic preterm labor or nonreassuring fetal testing. Bleeding may or may not be present. It is estimated that 50% of patients with abruption are already in established labor when the abruption occurs. Management includes maternal and fetal stabilization. If there is no evidence of fetal or maternal compromise, conservative management of pregnancy can be followed. Placenta previa (PP) and low-lying placenta can be correctly diagnosed by ultrasound with greater than 95% accuracy. Neither was present on ultrasound in this patient. Most experts agree that the use of ultrasound is to exclude placenta previa and not to diagnose placental abruption. Cervical laceration or trauma may be considered in the differential diagnosis of third-trimester bleeding but usually does not present with such a large blood loss. A succenturiate lobe of the placenta is associated with postpartum hemorrhage from retained placenta. Rupture of membranes is not usually associated with significant blood loss except in the presence of PP, PA, or vasa previa.

2 A 34-year-old gravida 2, para 1001 at 31 weeks' gestation with known placenta previa presents to Labor and Delivery with vaginal bleeding and contractions. Antenatal course is remarkable for one previous episode of vaginal bleeding during the second trimester. The patient reports she soaked two pads while at work. She reports good fetal movement. She denies any leakage of fluid. She denies feeling lightheaded or dizzy. Blood pressure is 100/65 and heart rate is 69 beats per minute. Fetal heart rate tracing is reassuring. On tocodynamometer, contractions are recorded every 7–10 minutes. On speculum examination, there is no active bleeding. The patient's hemoglobin is 11 g/dL. The most appropriate management is

A. Primary cesarean delivery
B. Biophysical profile
C. Intravenous (IV) tocolysis with magnesium sulfate
D. Amniocentesis for fetal lung maturity
E. Subcutaneous terbutaline

C The usual presentation of placenta previa (PP) is sudden, painless vaginal bleeding, occurring most commonly in the late second or third trimester. The earlier the initial bleeding episode, the worse is the overall prognosis for the pregnancy. Approximately 50% of patients with placenta previa will develop vaginal bleeding with or without uterine contractions. Despite expectant management, 20% deliver by 32 weeks' gestation. It is this subgroup that accounts for about 70% of the perinatal morbidity associated with this condition. Placenta previa is diagnosed by ultrasound more than 95% of the time. The timing and route of delivery depend on gestational age, amount of blood loss, and condition of the pregnant woman and fetus. If the patient is at or close to term, delivery is appropriate. A patient with heavy bleeding and evidence of hemodynamic compromise should promptly undergo cesarean delivery. In patients remote from term, expectant management is an option. A patient who is in the early third trimester and is hemodynamically stable with uterine activity is a candidate for tocolysis. Beta-mimetics should be avoided because they may aggravate the maternal hypotension from hypovolemia. In addition, the maternal tachycardia that occurs as a side effect of the drug may further confuse the clinical picture. Therefore, magnesium sulfate is considered a better choice. The patient at risk for preterm delivery should be given antenatal steroids to benefit the neonatal outcome. A patient at 34 weeks' gestation who is hemodynamically stable, having had one or more episodes of vaginal bleeding during pregnancy, would be a candidate for amniocentesis for assessment of fetal lung maturity. Cesarean delivery should follow a mature result. A stable patient, for example, at 32 weeks' gestation with known placenta previa and minimal vaginal bleeding with decreased fetal movement, would be a candidate for a biophysical profile.

11

Congenital Anomalies

Dana Gossett
Edith Gurewitsch

1 You receive a phone call from your obstetric patient regarding her triple screen (multiple serum marker) results. She is a 19-year-old gravida 1 para 0 now at 18 weeks' gestation. You review her triple screen results, which are shown below:

AFP: 0.61 MoM
hCG: 0.50 MoM
uE3: 0.39 MoM

You advise the patient that:

A. She needs to come in for a detailed anatomic ultrasound to rule out a neural tube defect or abdominal wall defect.

B. She should not be concerned about the results, as they probably reflect wrong dates. When all three values are low, the pregnancy is usually earlier than was believed.

C. Although her results are not typical, her age should make any kind of genetic abnormality unlikely. She is not old enough to merit further workup such as amniocentesis.

D. Her results are concerning for aneuploidy and she should come in for a detailed ultrasound and amniocentesis.

E. Her results are concerning for genetic or structural abnormality. She should come in for a detailed ultrasound, and if that is abnormal she may need an amniocentesis.

D Neural tube defects and abdominal wall defects result in elevated maternal serum AFP. This results from leakage of fetal protein into the amniotic fluid and subsequently into the maternal circulation. The result shown is not consistent with a neural tube or abdominal wall defect. In fact, the three markers do not increase together. AFP and uE3 tend to increase as gestational age increases, while hCG peaks around 12 weeks' gestation and begins to decline thereafter. A result suggestive of earlier dates would have low AFP and uE3, but elevated hCG. The risk for aneuploidy does increase with age. Statistically speaking, however, most aneuploid fetuses are born to women under 35. An abnormal serum marker result should not be ignored because of the patient's age. When all three values of the serum marker screen are low, and particularly when values are less than 0.4 MoM, the clinician should suspect trisomy 18. Because trisomy 18 may demonstrate no sonographic evidence of anatomic abnormality, or isolated growth restriction, amniocentesis should be offered even if the sonogram is normal. The patient should be offered amniocentesis for karyotype.

2 A 27-year-old gravida 2 para 0010 presents for her routine anatomy sonogram at a gestation of 19 weeks. She is found to have a singleton fetus, variable presentation, normal placentation, and mildly elevated amniotic fluid volume. Survey of the fetal anatomy reveals a "double bubble" sign, but no other abnormalities. You tell her all of the following *except:*

A. She is likely to develop polyhydramnios due to decreased fluid absorption by the fetal gut.

B. She should initiate antenatal fetal testing at 28 weeks' gestation.

C. Isolated duodenal atresia has a very good prognosis after surgical correction.

D. She should be offered amniocentesis for karyotyping.

E. She should have a fetal echocardiogram.

D Polyhydramnios is an almost universal finding with duodenal atresia. There is no indication for antenatal testing for isolated duodenal atresia, even if polyhydramnios is present. She should, however, be counseled about the risks of preterm labor due to polyhydramnios, and should be made aware of signs and symptoms of preterm labor. When duodenal atresia is isolated, quality of life after postnatal surgical repair should be excellent. As nearly 30% of fetuses with duodenal atresia have trisomy 21, she should be offered karyotype analysis. Approximately 20% of fetuses with duodenal atresia have associated cardiac defects. She should be offered fetal echocardiography.

3 You are covering the Labor and Delivery suite when a 31-year-old gravida 3 para 2002 at 29 weeks' gestation presents complaining of contractions. She has had intermittent prenatal care with your group; her last visit was at 21 weeks' gestation. She has not yet had a sonogram, as she missed her scheduled anatomic survey. As you perform a quick sonogram to confirm fetal presentation, you note free-floating loops of bowel in the amniotic cavity. There is no radiologist in house. To better define the diagnosis you should attempt to do all of the following *except:*

A. Visualize a membranous covering over the herniated loops of bowel sonographically.

B. Determine via sonography if the defect is in the midline, or to the left or right of the umbilical cord insertion.

C. Determine via sonography if other abdominal contents are herniating through the defect, such as liver.

D. Determine the position of the fetal heart (situs) sonographically.

E. Perform an amniocentesis for karyotype.

E A membranous covering is diagnostic of omphalocele, which has a different and sometimes far worse prognosis than gastroschisis. Failure to see an abdominoperitoneal membrane is suggestive of gastroschisis, although there is always a concern that it could be a ruptured omphalocele. In omphaloceles, the umbilical cord inserts into the hernia sac, in the midline. In gastroschisis, the defect is almost universally to the right of midline. The presence of liver evisceration in omphalocele is an ominous finding; in gastroschisis, the amount of bowel exposed to amniotic fluid can predict the amount of damage (stricturing) that may occur. If the heart is malpositioned (ectopia cordis) due to massive herniation into an omphalocele, the prognosis for the fetus is significantly worse. Until the diagnosis of omphalocele has been made with some certainty, karyotype analysis should be reserved. While up to 5% of cases of omphaloceles are associated with aneuploidy, there is no significant association with gastroschisis.

4 A patient presents for her second prenatal visit with you at 16 weeks' gestation. At her first visit, at 10 weeks' gestation, you were unable to auscult Doppler fetal heart tones, but attributed this to her obesity. Today, you are able to faintly detect a fetal heart rate in the 60s. It is not possible to monitor the fetus, due to gestational age and maternal obesity. You send her for an ultrasound, which shows an active fetus, a normal amniotic fluid volume, and confirms a fetal heart rate in the 60s. The limited sonographic evaluation of the heart is normal for gestational age. To manage the fetal bradycardia you:

A. Advise her that the fetus is bradycardic, which is evidence of distress, but that at this gestational age nothing can be done.

B. Schedule her for fetal monitoring every 2 weeks.

C. Schedule her for an anatomic sonogram and fetal echocardiogram at 20 weeks.

D. Start the patient on dcxamethasone therapy.

E. Perform an amniocentesis for karyotypic analysis.

C With an active fetus, the bradycardia is unlikely to represent an agonal rhythm. It is more likely that the fetus has complete (third-degree) heart block. There is no utility in monitoring a previable fetus, and routine monitoring in fetuses with complete heart block can be difficult or impossible. To determine the cause of the heart block, she needs a fetal echocardiogram between 20 and 22 weeks' gestation. If there is no structural abnormality to explain the arrhythmia, the patient should be screened for anti-Ro and -La (SSA and SSB) antibodies. If the patient is found to have an immune cause for the fetal heart block (anti-Ro or -La antibodies,) then dexamethasone may reduce the damage to the fetal heart. These antibodies cross the placenta and cause inflammation and fibrosis on the fetal conducting sytem. Until the cause of the heart block has been established, however, steroids should not be initiated. Because as many as half of cases of complete heart block may be due to maternal antibodies, routine karyotypic analysis is not justified. If, however, there is an associated cardiac structural anomaly, the rate of aneuploidy is up to 4–5%, and amniocentesis should be offered.

12

Perinatal Infections

Dana Virgo
Brenda Ross

1 A 26-year-old woman gravida 2 para 1001, at 20-1/7 weeks' gestation with a previously uncomplicated pregnancy undergoes a routine obstetrical sonogram showing a growth-restricted fetus (EFW <10th percentile). For which fetal infections should this patient be screened?

A. HIV

B. Rubella, cytomegalovirus (CMV), and toxoplasmosis

C. Parvovirus B19

D. Group B *Streptococcus* (GBS)

B Up to 10% of cases of fetal growth restriction may be due to various fetal infections. Early growth restriction particularly is suspicious for an insult such as a viral, bacterial, protozoan, or spirochetal infection. Among viruses, both rubella and CMV are associated with intrauterine growth restriction. Congenital rubella infection may involve multiple organ systems, leading to ocular defects, cardiac abnormalities, sensorineural deafness, and encephalopathy. Mortality of infants with congenital rubella ranges from 5% to 35%. Diagnosis is made by identification of rubella-specific IgM in fetal blood obtained by cordocentesis. CMV, the most common congenital infection, may cause growth restriction, petechiae, hepatosplenomegaly, jaundice, microcephaly with periventricular calcifications, oligohydramnios, premature delivery, and chorioretinitis. Typically, ultrasonography is used to identify fetal anomalies characteristic of CMV infection, then amniocentesis and cordocentesis may be used to measure total and specific cytomegalovirus IgM antibodies and to detect the virus via polymerase chain reaction (PCR) or culture. Among protozoal infections, toxoplasmosis is most often associated with growth restriction. Toxoplasmosis also may cause hepatosplenomegaly, icterus, and anemia. To rule out toxoplasmosis, maternal IgM and IgG titers may be sent. PCR testing also may be performed on amniotic fluid specimens.

Pregnancies in women infected with HIV have an increased risk of growth restriction, but usually due to factors other than fetal infection with the virus. Universal screening of pregnant women for HIV is recommended; however, if this patient has not been screened previously, it would be appropriate to offer HIV screening now. Parvovirus B19 is primarily associated with fetal anemia and nonimmune hydrops fetalis and typically does not cause fetal growth restriction. It is diagnosed by measuring maternal IgM and IgG titers. GBS is a leading cause of pneumonia, sepsis, and meningitis in neonates, as well as chorioamnionitis during pregnancy, but is not associated with growth restriction. It is diagnosed in pregnancy via vaginal culture of the mother. The lower third of the vagina, the perineum near the introitus, and the perianal region should be sampled with a swab which should be cultured with selective medium. GBS colonization is common, found in about one-third of women. It also is intermittent, so it is most appropriate to obtain the vaginal culture close to term.

2 A 25-year-old woman at 37 weeks' gestation, with a known history of genital herpes, comes to the office complaining of a herpes outbreak. On examination, she is noted to have the characteristic vesicular lesions on her right inner thigh. You counsel her that:

A. She should be delivered by cesarean section to avoid the risk of neonatal infection.

B. She should immediately start valacyclovir treatment and expect a vaginal delivery if the lesions have cleared when she goes into labor.

C. Her risk of cervical virus shedding is low, so she may deliver vaginally.

C Approximately 1 in 7,500 live-born infants contracts herpes simplex virus (HSV) perinatally. The incidence of asymptomatic shedding of HSV in pregnancy is 10% after a first episode and 0.5% after a recurrent episode. Fetal infection with HSV can occur via three routes. Transplacental transmission and ascending infection from the cervix both occur antenatally. However, the most common route of congenital infection with HSV is direct contact with infectious maternal genital lesions during delivery. Congenital infections resulting from recurrent maternal infection are rare, accounting for less than 1% of fetal infections. The transplacental passage of protective maternal IgG antibody is believed to account for the low rate of transmission in the context of recurrent maternal infection. However, the majority of congenital infections ultimately produce disseminated or CNS disease, with a mortality rate of 60%. Therefore, women with active herpes lesions in the genital area at the time of labor should be delivered by cesarean section. HSV recurrences in the regions of the buttocks, thighs, and anus are associated with low rates of cervical virus shedding, so vaginal delivery is acceptable. In these cases, covering the area of the lesion with a dressing during labor is recommended. In the event of HSV recurrence in the third trimester, treatment with valacyclovir (500 mg twice daily) is recommended to accelerate clearance of the lesions. Valacyclovir suppression (500 mg daily) should be considered in women with frequent outbreaks during their pregnancies.

3 You deliver a full-term infant to a 22-year-old woman, gravida 2 para 1001, after an uncomplicated pregnancy. The infant is noted to be small for gestational age at birth. On examination, the infant is noted to have a fever, petechial rash, microcephaly, and hepatosplenomegaly. Microscopy of the infant's urine sediment reveals large nuclear inclusion-bearing cells. The pediatrician will be most interested in which maternal tests?

A. Varicella zoster IgG

B. Rubeola antibody titer

C. Cytomegalovirus IgM and IgG
D. HIV antibody (ELISA)

C Ten to 15% of infants with congenital cytomegalovirus (CMV) infection have clinically apparent disease; 90% of these infants develop sequelae. Manifestations in the neonate may include a petechial rash, hepatosplenomegaly, jaundice, microcephaly with periventricular calcifications, and growth restriction. Inspection of urine sediment will reveal large nuclear inclusion-bearing cells. This infant has several characteristic signs of congenital CMV infection.

Maternal testing for CMV is problematic. Most primary CMV infections are asymptomatic, so the majority are undiagnosed. Screening asymptomatic women for seroconversion is not recommended because distinguishing primary from secondary infection is difficult. Only 75% of individuals with primary CMV infection will have CMV IgM, while 10% of those with secondary infection also will have IgM. Additionally, there is no effective *in utero* therapy for CMV. In the event of evidence of congenital infection during pregnancy or after delivery, maternal serum testing for IgM and IgG is recommended, though these tests should be interpreted with caution. Amniotic fluid analysis may be performed using polymerase chain reaction (PCR) to detect viral antigen. In the event that cord blood is available, testing for cord serum IgM is useful as well.

Congenital varicella syndrome typically afflicts infants of mothers with primary varicella infection prior to 20 weeks' gestation. Its manifestations include cutaneous scars, limb-reduction anomalies, malformed digits, muscle atrophy, growth restriction, cataracts, chorioretinitis, micropthalmia, cortical atrophy, microcephaly, and retardation. Most women with a history of varicella infection will have varicella zoster IgG, so this testing is nonspecific.

No definitive evidence of teratogenic influence of rubeola (measles) virus exists. Infants born to infected mothers are at risk of neonatal infection due to transplacental transmission of the virus. Clinical diagnosis is reliable, but when a patient's presentation is atypical, serologic studies may be required. There is no evidence that HIV has teratogenic effects in the fetus.

4 You are called to Labor and Delivery to evaluate a 35-year-old woman, gravida 6 para 3114, at 35 weeks' gestation by her last menstrual period, who has not received any prenatal care. The patient reports active intravenous drug use. She is having uterine contractions every 5 minutes and her cervix is dilated 5 cm. You send prenatal laboratories, including a rapid HIV test, which returns with a positive result. You:

A. Start the patient on intravenous zidovudine with a 2-mg/kg bolus then 1 mg/kg per hour until delivery.

B. Perform an amniotomy to expedite delivery and treatment of the newborn with oral zidovudine.

C. Perform an urgent cesarean delivery to reduce the risk of vertical transmission of the virus.

A In 1994, the AIDS Clinical Trials Group 076 showed that administration of zidovudine (ZDV) during pregnancy and childbirth could reduce vertical transmission rates of HIV by two-thirds. Further studies have found that ZDV is efficacious in reducing transmission even in the context of advanced disease, low maternal CD4 cell counts, and prior use of ZDV therapy. It is therefore vitally important to offer this regimen to all HIV-infected pregnant women. The recommended regimen is 100 mg of ZDV orally, five times daily, during the antepartum period and intravenous ZDV (2-mg/kg bolus, then 1 mg/kg per hour) in labor. This patient received no prenatal care and has been on no antiretroviral medications. It is important to start her on intravenous ZDV expeditiously.

To decrease the risk of maternal–fetal transfusion, certain procedures should be avoided during labor, including fetal scalp blood sampling and use of fetal scalp electrodes. Amniotomy also should be avoided, as there is an association between vertical transmission and the duration of rupture of membranes. Delivery *en caul* may confer some protection to the infant from vertical transmission. In this case, expediting vaginal delivery by stimulation of labor or amniotomy should be avoided, to allow the administration of intravenous ZDV for at least 4 hours prior to delivery.

Avoidance of labor also may decrease the risk of transmission. Some studies have shown a decrease in the risk of vertical transmission when scheduled cesarean delivery is performed as opposed to vaginal delivery or unscheduled cesarean delivery. However, most of this evidence was compiled before the use of highly active antiretroviral therapy (HAART) and without data regarding maternal viral load. Whether scheduled cesarean delivery decreases vertical transmission rates in women on HAART or with low viral loads is unknown. The impact of the length of labor or of rupture of membranes on vertical transmission in unscheduled cesarean deliveries is also unknown. Maternal morbidity is higher with cesarean delivery than with vaginal delivery. Increases in maternal morbidity seem to be greatest in HIV-infected women with lower CD4 cell counts. In general, HIV-infected pregnant women should be counseled on the existing evidence and offered a choice between vaginal delivery and scheduled cesarean delivery. This particular patient is already in labor, which decreases the protection possibly conferred by cesarean delivery. Her viral load and CD4 count are unknown. The most protective action would be prompt administration of intravenous ZDV, followed by discussion of delivery plan with the patient.

5 You see a 30-year-old primigravida at 8-1/7 weeks' gestation pregnancy for her first obstetric visit. She tells you that she owns a cat. You counsel her as follows:

A. She should avoid contact with her cat during her pregnancy.

B. She should avoid contact with used cat litter and cat feces for the duration of her pregnancy.

C. She should be tested for *Toxoplasma* exposure by sending an IgG titer.

B The incidence of acute toxoplasmosis infection in pregnant U.S. women is 0.2–1.0%. Congenital toxoplasmosis occurs in 1–8/1,000 live births. Adults with the infection typically have contracted it via ingestion of undercooked or raw meat containing cysts, ingestion of food or water contaminated by feces of an infected cat, or handling material contaminated by feces from an infected cat. The most common manifestation of the infection in adults is a mononucleosis-like syndrome, including fatigue, malaise, cervical lymphadenopathy, and atypical lymphocytosis. In pregnancy, placental infection and subsequent fetal infection occur during the spreading phase of the parasitemia. The overall risk of fetal infection is 30–40%. The risk of vertical transmission increases with gestational age, though fetal morbidity and mortality rates are higher after early transmission. Infected neonates may demonstrate low birthweight, hepatosplenomegaly, icterus, and anemia. Long-term sequelae including visual loss, hearing loss, and psychomotor and mental retardation are common.

Approximately one-third of U.S. women carry *Toxoplasmosa* antibodies. Screening with IgG or IgM titers is not routine or necessary. Pregnant women with cat exposure should avoid handling cat feces or litter for the duration of their pregnancies. Serologic testing should be limited to women who present with symptoms of acute toxoplasmosis. Amniotic fluid testing using PCR also may be useful.

6 A 21-year-old woman, gravida 2 para 0010, at 37 weeks' gestation, calls your office because she has been exposed to chicken pox. She does not recall a history of the illness.

A. You send a varicella zoster IgG titer within 24–48 hours of exposure to assess her susceptibility to the virus.

B. You administer varicella zoster immune globulin within 72–96 hours of her exposure to prevent possible maternal–fetal transmission of the virus.

C. You advise her that immediate induction of labor is recommended to avoid the risk of maternal–fetal transmission of the virus.

D. You recommend immediate vaccination using attenuated live vaccine.

A The incidence of varicella in pregnancy is approximately 0.7 per 1,000 pregnancies. This low frequency is related to the high likelihood of exposure in childhood. When a pregnant woman without a known history of chicken pox is exposed to a person with noncrusted varicella zoster virus (VZV) lesions, an IgG titer should be obtained within 24–48 hours of the exposure. The virus is rarely isolated from crusted lesions, so such an exposure carries a much lower risk. In most cases, VZV IgG will be present, indicating prior immunity. In the absence of IgG, the woman is susceptible.

The incubation period for the virus is 13–17 days. Primary varicella infection tends to be more severe in adults, and particularly during pregnancy. Pregnant women have an increased risk of varicella pneumonia, with a mortality rate approaching 40% in the absence of therapy. Signs or symptoms of varicella pneumonia should be managed aggressively in pregnancy.

If maternal infection occurs within 5 days of delivery, hematogenous transplacental viral transfer may cause significant neonatal morbidity, incurring mortality rates between 10% and 30%. Sufficient antibody transfer to protect the fetus apparently requires 5 days after the onset of the maternal rash. Women who develop chicken pox near term should be observed for signs of labor. Tocolysis should be initiated if labor begins before the fifth day of the maternal infection. Induction of labor should be avoided in susceptible women with recent exposure to the virus. If delivery occurs prior to the fifth day of maternal infection, the neonate should receive varicella immune globulin.

ACOG currently recommends the administration of varicella zoster immune globulin (VZIG) to susceptible, exposed pregnant women. Given within 72–96 hours of exposure, VZIG is 60–80% effective in preventing maternal infection. Dosing of VZIG is one vial (125 Us) per 10 kg body weight with a maximal dose of five vials. Alternatively, prophylactic acyclovir (800 mg orally five times daily for 5–7 days) may be given. There is no evidence that either practice decreases the risk of maternal–fetal transmission of the virus in the event of maternal infection.

An attenuated live vaccine was approved by the FDA in 1995. Two doses, given 4–8 weeks apart, are recommended for adults without a history of varicella infection. The vaccine should be offered to all susceptible women of reproductive age. Use of the vaccine is contraindicated in women who are pregnant or immunocompromised.

13

Endocrine Disorders of Pregnancy

Janice Falls

1 A 39-year-old para 0100 presents to the emergency department with abdominal pain and vaginal spotting. An ultrasound is performed and the patient is newly diagnosed with an intrauterine pregnancy at 29 weeks' gestation, with an anterior placenta. The patient reports a weight gain of approximately 10 lbs and reports no urinary symptoms. She has eaten nothing for the last 8 hours. Her history includes a fetal death *in utero* from a probable "cord accident" at 34 weeks' gestation. The patient's labs are as follows: hematocrit 34.1%, platelets 261,000, sodium 134, potassium 4.6, glucose 191, AST 30, ALT 22, bilirubin (total) 0.6, serum osmolality 289, and amylase and lipase are within normal limits. After fully assessing this patient, the optimal management would include:

A. Encourage the patient to follow up in clinic for a glucose challenge test.

B. Send a glycosylated hemoglobin (HbA1C) and have the patient follow up in clinic.

C. Start an American Diabetes Association (ADA) diet and low-dose insulin therapy for glucose management, and have the patient follow up in clinic.

D. Start an ADA diet, begin recording of fasting and postprandial glucose, and follow up for a test of fasting blood glucose.

E. Immediately hospitalize the patient for further paneling and management of her diabetes.

D Initially managing a patient with pregestational or gestational diabetes can be difficult. If a patient presents with hyperglycemia prior to 20 weeks' gestation, she more than likely has pregestational diabetes (PDM). Gestational diabetes (GDM) is usually a disorder of late gestation. The glucose challenge test is a screening test, optimally given at 26–28 weeks' gestation. Accuracy is increased if given in a fasting state. The test would not be indicated at this time, as the patient has already demonstrated hyperglycemia. However, a fasting glucose would better define this patient's diabetes and should be considered. If the value is greater than 126 mg/dL, a glucose tolerance test (GTT) may be indicated, or the patient could be managed as GDM while paneling ensued. If the level is less than 126 mg/dL, then a GTT should be performed.

Hemoglobin A1C is a good indicator of a patient's serum glucose values over the previous 6–8 weeks. This is especially important during embryogenesis, as the rate of fetal malformations is highest during that time. As this patient has long since passed organogenesis, an HbA1C would have less relevance now. However, it would provide information of glucose control and a general indication as to how poorly managed her glucose levels have been. A HbA1C greater than 10% during organogenesis is associated with significant risk of fetal malformations. If the levels are within normal range, the risk appears to be similar to that of a nondiabetic woman.

The patient's daily serum glucose values are not known, and in this setting, starting insulin would not be indicated, as the patient has not had proper counseling and training for self-injections, and the dosing would be difficult to determine based on one glucose level. She should be paneled (recording fasting, and 1- or 2-hour postprandial glucose values) to better guide insulin dosing if it is in fact required. An ADA diet should be started as well. Diet recommendations range from 1,800 to 2,400 kcal (usually 2,100 to 2,200 kcal), including 15–20% protein, 50–60% carbohydrates, and up to 20%

fat. It takes approximately 48 hours for an ADA diet to reflect associated glucose levels. After this, insulin therapy, if needed, can be started.

Hospitalizing the patient can be considered, though she has no evidence of ketoacidosis or other metabolic deficiency. While she may not be the optimal patient to send home because of her status of no prior prenatal care and history of a fetal death, it would be reasonable to give explicit instructions on checking her glucose levels and providing her with good follow-up in clinic.

2 A 27-year-old gravida 4, para 2012 at 35 weeks' gestation presents to the emergency department with confusion, dizziness, nausea, and vomiting. The patient is unable to give an accurate history of onset of symptoms. Her past medical history is significant for type 1 diabetes, diagnosed at 16 years of age. Her medications include Humalog and NPH. A prior HbA1C was known to be 10.1%. The patient's vitals include temperature of 37.6°C, blood pressure 88/39 mm Hg, pulse 111, respiration 26. She is diaphoretic. Laboratory values include hemoglobin 9.4, sodium 129, potassium 4.9, glucose 381, serum ketones greater than 1:4, arterial cord gas pH 7.22, P_{CO_2} 30, P_{O_2} 92, HCO_3 14, base excess −6. Urine has 3+ ketones, 3+ glucose. The first thing you do to stabilize the patient is:

A. Start PO hydration, check glucose levels every 1–2 hours, providing regular insulin subcutaneously (SC) as needed.

B. Begin vigorous IV hydration, using dextrose 5% (D5) lactated Ringers solution with insulin drip, and start broad-spectrum antibiotics, while monitoring glucose and electrolytes.

C. Begin vigorous IV hydration using normal saline (NS) with insulin drip, and assess for infection, while monitoring glucose and electrolytes.

D. Begin D5$\frac{1}{2}$ NS at 125 cc per hour, an antiemetic, and an H2 blocker, and monitor glucose levels.

C Risk factors for diabetic ketoacidosis (DKA) include new-onset diabetes; pulmonary, urinary, or soft tissue infections; cocaine use; and poor glucose control. Maternal plasma glucose and ketones are readily transported to the fetus, which may precipitate DKA in the fetus as well. In the setting of DKA, the patient's initial management is critical to her well-being, as she has become hyperosmolar and hypovolemic.

Insulin therapy is essential in managing this patient, as DKA is caused by and results in impaired insulin action. Supplemental insulin is needed to increase glucose uptake. Usually a continuous infusion of insulin is used, though injections may be given instead. An IV bolus of 10–20 U should be given initially, followed by an infusion rate of 5–10 U per hour, to be adjusted according to glucose levels.

Intravenous fluids should be started, providing 1 L of normal saline in the first hour, then running fluids in at least 250 cc per hour thereafter. The patient may require more than 5 L in the first 24 hours. Normal saline should be used, as the patient is greatest risk of severe hyponatremia. It is also important that the sodium levels not be corrected too quickly, because of potential for seizures and neurologic dysfunction. The volume deficit should be repleted within 12–24 hours, and the sodium deficit should be replaced in approximately 6 hours. When serum glucose falls below 250 mg/dL, then D5 fluids may be added.

If the patient is hyperkalemic, an ECG should be performed, and potassium should not be started until good urine output ensues. If potassium is normal or low, along with an ECG, the patient should be started on 20 mEq per hour of potassium (after the first liter of NS is in), as long as she is not oliguric. In the setting of oliguria, potassium should be started at 10 mEq per hour, and increased to 20 mEq per hour once urine output is established. Potassium levels should be checked frequently, and dosing adjusted accordingly. The patient will have an overall potassium deficit and may require replacement for up to 1 week following the inciting event. Bicarbonate and phosphorous should be monitored as well, and repleted only as needed.

Infection is often the precipitating event causing a patient to develop DKA. Antibiotic coverage can have a significant impact on DKA if there is an infectious etiology. Broad-spectrum antibiotics should be started if an infectious source is suspected.

3 A 36-year-old gravida 2, para 1001 at 39 weeks' gestation presents in labor with a cervical exam of 7 cm. The patient has type 2 diabetes, and is on a total of 66 U of NPH and 52 U of regular insulin daily. She has had difficulty with her insurance and has been unable to take her normal insulin doses for the last 2 days. A recent HbA1C was 4.1%. The estimated fetal weight is 3,400 g. Intrapartum, the patient's glucose levels range from 150 to 262 mg/dL. The patient progresses to full dilatation and begins pushing. When the fetus delivers, it is at greatest risk for which of the following:

A. Hypoglycemia secondary to increased production of fetal insulin

B. Hypoglycemia secondary to increased production of maternal insulin

C. Macrosomia and possible increased head circumference resulting in a difficult delivery

D. Macrosomia and possible need for cesarean section

A Serum glucose levels should be tightly controlled during the immediate antepartum, and the intrapartum period. This patient appears to have had good glucose control during her pregnancy, as her HbA1C is within normal range and estimated fetal weight is appropriate. However, during the intrapartum period she has had poor control. The greatest risk to the fetus in this setting is hypoglycemia. Up to 40% of infants of diabetic mothers will develop hypoglycemia in the first few hours after birth.

Infant hypoglycemia is due to poor maternal glycemic control during pregnancy, up to 48 hours prior to delivery, and from elevated intrapartum maternal glucose levels. Maternal hyperglycemia stimulates increased production of maternal insulin. Insulin, however, is too large to cross the placenta. Glucose crosses the placenta, and in the case of hyperglycemia, it will increase fetal insulin production. After delivery, when the umbilical cord is cut, the fetus no longer is exposed to the high glucose load and will subsequently develop hypoglycemia. The resultant hypoglycemia in a newborn, if severe, can cause seizures, coma, brain damage, and death. This patient is at increased risk for fetal hypoglycemia because she has not taken her regular insulin for 2 days and her intrapartum levels are markedly elevated. Optimal maternal glucose control includes euglycemia for approximately 48 hours before delivery, including the intrapartum period. Patients should have intrapartum glucose levels ranging between 60 and 100 mg/dL.

If the fetus has had significant antepartum hyperglycemic exposure, even in the setting of intrapartum euglycemia, hypoglycemia may occur due to fetal islet cell hypertrophy and chronic hyperinsulinemia. It is important for infants of diabetic mothers to have glucose levels checked frequently after birth.

Macrosomia, defined as fetal weight greater than the 90th percentile, or 4,000 g, is a significant risk for infants of poorly controlled diabetic mothers. However, this patient appears to have had good antepartum glycemic control with a low HbA1C. The fetus also has an estimated fetal weight within normal limits. In the setting of fetal macrosomia in poorly controlled maternal diabetes, it is usually the abdominal circumference (AC) that is enlarged secondary to subcutaneous fat deposits from fetal hyperinsulinemia. The head circumference (HC) is not significantly affected by diabetes. The HC:AC ratio decreases with fetal macrosomia.

4 All of the following congenital malformations are associated with poorly controlled pregestational diabetes *except:*

A. Cardiac asymmetric septal hypertrophy

B. Situs inversus

C. Caudal regression syndrome

D. Tracheoesophageal fistula

E. Polydactyly

E Women with gestational, type 1, or type 2 diabetes are at increased risk for congenital malformations when compared to normal pregnancies, though type 1 and type 2 diabetes put a patient at greater risk of malformations than does gestational diabetes. Up to 50% of perinatal mortality can be attributed to congenital malformations. Maternal hyperglycemia is believed to be the primary cause of these malformations, though hypoglycemia and hyperketonemia have been implicated.

Congenital malformations associated with poorly controlled diabetes are:

- CNS—Anencephaly, holoprosenscephaly, microcephaly, spina bifida, encephalocele, and meningomyelocele
- Cardiovascular—Transposition of the great vessels, ventricular and atrial septal defects, asymmetric septal hypertrophy, hypoplastic left ventricle, situs inversus, and aortic anomalies
- Gastrointestinal—Tracheoesophageal fistula, bowel atresia, small bowel stricture, imperforate anus
- Genitourinary—Absent kidneys (Potter's syndrome), polycystic kidneys, double ureter
- Skeletal—Caudal regression syndrome

Polydactyly does not appear to be associated with diabetes in pregnancy.

5 A 31-year-old nullipara at 28 weeks' gestation presents for her first prenatal visit. The patient states she has lost approximately 5 lbs over the last few weeks. She is thin, mildly diaphoretic, and appears agitated. On further workup she is found to be hyperthyroid. If the patient has had poor control of her thyroid disease throughout her pregnancy, she would be at greatest risk for developing which of the following?

A. Dry, coarse skin

B. Reflexive bradycardia

C. Preeclampsia

D. Polycythemia

E. Hypocalcemia

C Hyperthyroidism in pregnancy, if not controlled, can lead to thyroid storm, which can be life-threatening to the mother and fetus. Poorly controlled hyperthyroidism in pregnancy can result in maternal preeclampsia, congestive heart failure, thyroid storm, preterm labor and delivery, and fetal intrauterine growth restriction and stillbirth. Classic presenting signs and symptoms of maternal hyperthyroidism include heat intolerance; palpitations; diarrhea; tachycardia; exophthalmos;

thyromegaly; onycholysis; moist, warm skin; anemia; and difficulty gaining weight.

Preeclampsia is associated with hyperthyroidism, though the mechanism is not known. A patient who has been diagnosed with hyperthyroidism should be treated with propylthiouracil (PTU) (or carbimazole) even in the absence of symptoms. There is a higher rate of minor fetal anomalies associated with untreated or inadequately treated hyperthyroidism. Beta-blockers (i.e., propranolol) can be added if needed for further maternal cardiovascular management.

Tests to diagnose thyroid dysfunction in pregnancy include primarily thyroid-stimulating hormone (TSH) and free T4 (unbound, FT4). These tests should be performed in the first trimester if possible. If results are within normal limits after starting PTU, they do not need to be checked again until once each in the second and third trimesters. If the results are abnormal, then they should be checked every 3–4 weeks until the levels are within the normal range.

Mild hypercalcemia is also associated with hyperthyroidism, especially in the setting of Graves' disease. With hyperthyroidism, there is increased bone resorption, resulting in high-normal to mild hypercalcemia, and also hypercalciuria. The mildly elevated levels of serum and urine calcium usually pose no threat to the mother or fetus.

14

Hypertensive Disorders of Pregnancy

Lisa Soule
Frank Witter

1 A 17-year-old nullipara registers at 16 weeks' gestation with a blood pressure of 100/60. At 38 weeks' gestation, she is seen in the office with a blood pressure of 146/94 and trace proteinuria. She is sent to Labor and Delivery for further evaluation, where, on overnight observation, she is noted to have persistent pressures above 140/90. A 24-hour urine protein determination is 160 mg. Her diagnosis is

A. Mild preeclampsia
B. Pregnancy-induced hypertension
C. Chronic hypertension
D. Normal third-trimester blood pressures

B The diagnosis of pregnancy-induced hypertension is made by blood pressures higher than 140/90 first diagnosed after 20 weeks' gestation, in the absence of proteinuria greater than 300 mg on 24-hour collection, and without evidence of severe preeclampsia. Had this patient's proteinuria been over 300 mg (or greater than 1+ on urine dip), she would meet criteria for mild preeclampsia. Chronic hypertension is diagnosed based on blood pressures above 140/90 prior to 20 weeks' gestation or a diagnosis of hypertension made before pregnancy. While blood pressure does increase in the third trimester, pressures over 140/90 observed on two assessments 6 hours apart are not normal.

2 A 34-year-old gravida 3, para 1011 with a previous pregnancy delivered vaginally after induction of labor for preeclampsia at term is admitted at 33-3/7 weeks' gestation with blood pressures of 144/90 and 152/96 over several hours of monitoring. She has 440 mg of protein on a 24-hour urine collection. Her hematocrit is 34.2% and her platelets are 212,000. Her cervix is long, closed, and high, and she is not contracting. After 36 hours of conservative management, she complains of a headache that is not relieved with Tylenol. Repeat labs include a hematocrit of 38.0% and platelets of 98,000. Her blood pressure is 156/98 and she has 2+ proteinuria. Which criterion of severe preeclampsia is evident?

A. Blood pressure > 140/90

B. Proteinuria > 1+

C. Platelets < 100

D. Hemoconcentration (rising hematocrit)

C Blood pressure criteria for severe preeclampsia require systolic pressures of 160 or greater or diastolic pressures of 110 or greater. Proteinuria must be more than 5 g on a 24-hour collection or 3+ or greater on a urine dip. Platelets <100,000 are one of the laboratory criteria for severe preeclampsia, others being a new onset of creatinine of > 1.2 mg/dL, and AST ≥ 70 U/L. While hemoconcentration is frequently seen in severe preeclampsia, it is not a criterion for diagnosis. Symptoms of severe preeclampsia include altered consciousness, headache, scotomata, blurred vision, pulmonary edema, and epigastric or right-upper-quadrant pain.

3 Which patient does *not* have a significant risk factor for development of preeclampsia?

A. A 34-year-old para 2002 with prior uncomplicated pregnancies who is carrying triplets

B. A 16-year-old nullipara whose sister had preeclampsia

C. A 28-year-old para 1021 with a prior uncomplicated pregnancy who smokes one pack of cigarettes a day

D. A 33-year-old nullipara with class B diabetes

C Risk factors for preeclampsia include multiple gestation; family history of preeclampsia; age extremes (<20 or >40); nulliparity; presence of diabetes, lupus, renal disease, or chronic hypertension; previous history of preeclampsia/eclampsia. Smoking is actually associated with a decreased incidence of preeclampsia.

4 A 22-year-old gravida 2, para 0102 develops severe preeclampsia by blood pressure criteria at 35-6/7 weeks' gestation. Her cervix is 2 cm dilated, 80% effaced, and the fetal head is at −2 station. She is contracting irregularly. Her blood pressure on $MgSO_4$ is 142/92. Her lab values are normal and her urine output is 75–125 cc per hour. She denies headache, scotomata, or right-upper-quadrant pain. Her management should be

A. Immediate delivery by cesarean section

B. Expectant management

C. Discontinuation of $MgSO_4$ and transfer to the antenatal unit

D. Induction of labor with pitocin

D A patient with severe preeclampsia at more than 34 weeks' gestation should be delivered. $MgSO_4$ should be continued until 24 hours postpartum. In a stable patient with a favorable cervix and/or spontaneous contractions, immediate operative delivery is not necessary, but delivery should be expeditious.

5 A 17-year-old nullipara is diagnosed with preeclampsia at 30-3/7 weeks' gestation. Her maximal blood pressure has been 144/94 and her 24-hour urine protein is 500 mg. After review of the patient's labs, which are normal, and determination that she is asymptomatic, the decision is made to manage her conservatively. She is admitted to the inpatient antepartum floor, where her management should *not* include:

A. Bedrest

B. Weekly fetal growth sonograms

C. Blood pressure measurement every 4 hours

D. Biweekly CBC and LFTs

B Expectant management includes all of the measures above except weekly growth sonograms. Growth sonograms should not be undertaken more frequently than every 2–3 weeks because of the margin of error of the measurement. Additional components of expectant management include daily checks of urine output, symptomatology, deep tendon reflexes and fetal movement, 24-hour urine protein determinations every other day, and weekly to twice-weekly NSTs and/or biophysical profiles.

6 A 33-year-old gravida 8, para 4034 unregistered patient is brought in to the hospital seizing. Her blood pressure is 160/104. Estimated gestational age (EGA) is unknown, but her fundal height is 35 cm. Appropriate management would include all of the following measures *except*:

A. Immediate cesarean section

B. $MgSO_4$ loaded at 6 g over 20 minutes, then 2 g per hour, with an additional bolus of 2 g over 5–20 minutes if the patient seizes again

C. Total fluid restriction of 125 cc per hour and airway management

D. Treatment with hydralazine or labetolol for diastolic blood pressure of 105 or higher

A It is important to stabilize the patient before initiating delivery. While fetal bradycardia may occur in the face of maternal seizures, recovery is usually seen once the maternal condition is treated, and it is preferrable to allow the fetus time to recover *in utero* rather than delivering emergently. Persistent fetal bradycardia may signal placental abruption, however, and emergent cesarian should then be undertaken. Preeclamptic and eclamptic patients on magnesium are at increased risk of pulmonary edema, so fluid management should be rigorous and adequate oxygenation should be optimized. Whether or not seizures are occurring, diastolic pressures above 105 should be decreased with medical therapy.

7 A 35-year-old gravida 6, para 2123 registers for prenatal care at 11 weeks' gestation. Her registration blood pressure is 150/98. She had been treated with Captopril prior to her last pregnancy, was on Aldomet during her last pregnancy, but had not returned for medical follow-up until initiating prenatal care for the current pregnancy. As her pregnancy progresses, her pressures rise to 160/108. Appropriate medical management includes all *except*:

A. Hydralazine

B. Methyldopa (Aldomet)

C. Labetolol

D. Captopril

D The first-line treatment when antihypertensives are initiated during pregnancy is methyldopa, which is a centrally acting adrenergic inhibitor, or labetolol, an alpha- and beta-blocker. Hydralazine, a peripheral vasodilator, is a useful second-line agent, often used in combination with methyldopa or labetolol. ACE inhibitors, such as Captopril, should not be used in pregnancy because they are associated with fetal death *in utero* and neonatal renal failure.

8 A 42-year-old gravida 6, para 2032 has been hospitalized for 1 week with mild preeclampsia. She has been managed conservatively and is now at 31-6/7 weeks' gestation. She complains of new onset of right-upper-quadrant pain, and her morning labs show a drop in her platelets to 86,000, and newly elevated AST of 74 and ALT of 68. Which of the following statements is false?

A. She has met criteria for HELLP syndrome on the basis of elevated liver function tests and thrombocytopenia.

B. HELLP syndrome is invariably associated with blood pressures greater than 160/110.

C. She should be delivered expeditiously.

D. Severe thrombocytopenia may be treated with 10 mg dexamethasone IM or IV every 12 hours until platelets exceed 100,000.

B The diagnosis of HELLP requires platelet count <100,000; hemolysis as demonstrated by LDH > 600 U/L, bilirubin of 1.2 mg/dL or greater or by peripheral smear; or by elevated liver function tests, with AST $\geq$ 70. HELLP may present in the absence of any blood pressure elevations, in up to 20% of cases, or in association with mild preeclampsia in 30%. Delivery should be initiated regardless of gestational age, unless thrombocytopenia is the only finding, in which case delivery may be delayed to administer antenatal steroids if EGA is < 28 weeks.

15

Cardiopulmonary Disorders of Pregnancy

Songhai Barclift
Ernest Graham

1 What is the most common type of heart disease encountered in pregnancy?

A. Arrhythmia

B. Congenital heart disease

C. Cardiovascular disease

D. Hypertensive heart disease

B Heart disease is one of the major causes of maternal mortality, accounting for 6–8% of maternal deaths. Congenital heart disease accounts for more than half of the heart disease encountered in reproductive age women. Advances in surgical techniques have allowed more women with congenital lesions to reach reproductive age. Mitral valve prolapse is the most common lesion seen.

Commonly corrected congenital lesions will not adversely affect pregnancy. However, there is a 4% occurrence of fetal congenital heart lesions when the mother has a history of congenital heart disease. A fetal echocardiogram is recommended.

Hypertension is common in pregnancy, but hypertensive heart disease is a complication of longstanding hypertension. Women of reproductive age usually have not developed this complication.

Cardiovascular disease in pregnancy is uncommon mainly because reproductive-age patients usually have not developed severe vascular disease. When it is encountered, persons should be followed by a cardiologist for maximum medical management before pregnancy occurs.

Many women complain of palpitations, but arrhythmia is not commonly diagnosed. A prolonged Halter monitoring can be done to detect potentially lethal arrhythmias.

2 What are some symptoms during pregnancy that are more likely to indicate serious heart disease?

A. Systolic heart murmur
B. Worsening dyspnea on exertion
C. Pedal edema
D. Palpitations

B Many cardiac-related symptoms encountered in normal pregnancy mimic heart disorders in the nonpregnant state (see A2). Most of the time these symptoms are a result of the significant but physiologic cardiac and endocrine changes in pregnancy. Of the symptoms listed, worsening dyspnea is the most worrisome. It indicates a progressive, *uncompensated* cardiac or pulmonary disorder. In addition, chest pain, syncope, diastolic murmur, cyanosis, and jugular venous distention should all be thoroughly investigated.

The workup should include an electrocardiogram, cardiac enzymes, cardiac stress test, and echocardiogram as needed. The electrocardiogram changes that occur in normal pregnancy during the third trimester are left axis deviation, nonspecific ST segment changes in the inferior leads, and altered voltage.

3 In patients diagnosed with pulmonary hypertension, which period is *not* associated with increased maternal mortality?

A. Conception
B. Labor and delivery
C. Postpartum
D. Post-epidural anesthesia

A Pulmonary hypertension is mean pulmonary artery pressures > 24 mm Hg at rest and > 35 mm Hg with exertion. It can present as a primary disorder in which the etiology is unknown, or it can be a secondary complication of cardiopulmonary disease. When it is present during pregnancy, it can pose severe maternal and fetal risk.

The maternal mortality rate is 30%. Maternal morbidity can occur at all stages, but the hemodynamic changes that occur in the third trimester, during labor, and postpartum are more likely to result in maternal mortality. Since severe pulmonary hypertension is preload-dependent, every effort should be made to maximize preload and cardiac output. The preferred method of anesthesia is a regional block during the second stage. The hypotension associated with epidural is potentially lethal in severe cases. Laboring in the left lateral decubitus position offsets some of the decreased preload associated with uterine compression of the inferior vena cava. The fluid changes during a cesarean section may be a risk for increased mortality, so it should not be considered a safer alternative.

4 When investigating for pneumonia, a chest X-ray is contraindicated during pregnancy.

A. True

B. False

B **False.** Pneumonia is a common infection, affecting 0.1% of pregnancies. The diagnosis and prompt treatment of pneumonia is necessary to prevent the associated antepartum complications. There is a 44% risk of preterm labor and a 36% chance of preterm delivery. Moreover, serious complications such as adult respiratory distress syndrome and fetal distress can occur. Therefore a chest X-ray should not be delayed or deferred when attempting to diagnose pneumonia. Chest X-ray is associated with approximately 1.5 mrad and has not been shown to have any adverse affect on fetal development, but abdominal shielding is recommended.

5 Which one of the following is the best way to manage asthmatics during pregnancy?

A. Peak flows and questions regarding signs and symptoms at each prenatal visit

B. Pulmonary function test every trimester

C. Nonstress test twice a week during the third trimester

D. Empiric oral steroids for all severe asthmatics

A Asthma is a common disorder in reproductive-age women. It complicates 1% of all pregnancies. Pregnancy can have a variable effect on the severity of asthma. Moreover, pregnancies complicated by moderate to severe asthma are at increased risk for adverse pregnancy outcomes, probably secondary to chronic hypoxia, hypercapnia, and alkalosis.

Measurement of the peak expiratory flow rate is an inexpensive evaluation of functional status. Patients should therefore have access to a peak flow meter at home, where they can check their status daily. At each prenatal visit, patients should be screened for worsening symptoms. Treatment as well as indications for steroids, intubation, antihistamines, and antibiotics during pregnancy is the same as for the nonpregnant state. However, severe asthma that requires chronic steroid use or associated with chronic hypoxia can result in uteroplacental insufficiency. Only in this setting is antenatal testing helpful. The alkalosis associated with normal pregnancy can mask hypercapnia of hypoxia, making arterial blood gas measurements appear to be in the normal range.

16

Renal, Hepatic, and Gastrointestinal Disorders and Systemic Lupus Erythematosus in Pregnancy

Eli Rybak

For Questions 1–4, please refer to the following vignette.
A 38-year-old gravida 2 para 0101 presents to you for obstetric care at a gestational age of 7 weeks by her last menstrual period (LMP). She contends with chronic renal disease attributable to lupus nephritis, and she requires dialysis three times weekly.

1 Which of the following statements is *incorrect*?

- **A.** This patient has an increased risk of having a fetus with intrauterine growth restriction (IUGR), she has an increased risk of renal failure, and she assumes a higher risk of superimposed preeclampsia.
- **B.** The fetus of this patient is likely to develop the neonatal lupus syndrome.
- **C.** Antenatal management of this patient should include a 24-hour urine protein and creatinine clearance quantitation, a 20-week anomaly ultrasound followed by growth scans every 4 weeks, and close surveillance and fetal testing in the third trimester.

D. Dialysis sessions conducted late in pregnancy warrant continuous fetal heart monitoring.

B Systemic lupus erythematosus (SLE) is a multisystem rheumatologic disorder that typically afflicts reproductive-age women, particularly in the African-American community. When it occurs in a pregnant patient, SLE contributes to an increased risk of spontaneous abortion, IUGR, premature delivery, and intrauterine fetal death (IUFD). The presence of antiphospholipid antibodies potentiates the risk of fetal demise in the second trimester.

Chronic renal disease likewise associates with IUGR, preterm delivery, and increased fetal morbidity and mortality. Stratified into mild, moderate, and severe categories, chronic renal disease results from various pathologic processes including hypertension, diabetes, and SLE. Predictably, prenatal outcomes correlate with the degree of renal insufficiency.

Choice **B** is an incorrect statement. The neonatal lupus syndrome involves hematologic complications, cardiac abnormalities—particularly, complete heart block—and a transient rash. As stated in the chapter, however, this syndrome is rare. Susceptible neonates include only those born to mothers with antibodies to the Ro (SSA) or La (SSB) antigens. Of these, fewer than 3% develop congenital heart block. Accordingly, choice **B** is the correct response.

Choice **A** is a correct statement. Pregnant women suffering from chronic renal disease assume an elevated risk of IUGR, renal failure, and superimposed preeclampsia. Choice **C** is also true. Pregnant patients with preexisting renal disease, with or absent a concomitant diagnosis of SLE, are managed antenatally with baseline 24-hour screening values of urine protein and creatinine. In addition, close attention is paid both to the 20-week anomaly scan and to the results of third-trimester fetal testing. Growth scans every 4 weeks allow for the detection of IUGR. Fluid shifts common during dialysis may effect transient maternal hypotension and consequent uteroplacental insufficiency. Electrolyte abnormalities often ensue as well. Continuous fetal heart monitoring for dialysis late in pregnancy is therefore indicated.

2 A lupus flare in this patient can be distinguished from superimposed preeclampsia by all of the following criteria *except*:

A. Diminished complement levels

B. Elevated liver transaminase levels

C. Presence of red blood cell (RBC) casts in a urinalysis sample

D. Positive antinuclear antibody testing

E. Thrombocytopenia

E Fever, malaise, and the presence of lymphadenopathy suggest the presence of a lupus flare. Low C3 or C4 complement levels, RBC casts in a urine specimen, elevated anti-double-stranded DNA antibody titers, hemolytic anemia, and thrombocytopenia are characteristic findings in a lupus flare. The clinical and laboratory presentation of a lupus flare, however, often coincides with that of superimposed preeclampsia. These two clinical entities cannot be distinguished on the basis of criteria they share: hypertension, proteinuria, thrombocytopenia, and hyperuricemia. Thus, choice **E**, thrombocytopenia, is the correct answer. Distinguishing criteria, however, include complement levels (low in a lupus flare; normal in preeclampsia), liver function tests (normal in a lupus flare; potentially elevated in preeclampsia accompanied by the HELLP syndrome), and the presence of RBC casts in a urine specimen (suggestive of a lupus flare only). Additionally, positive antinuclear antibody testing is associated with SLE, not preeclampsia.

3 All of the following findings warrant a prompt lupus workup in an otherwise healthy pregnant patient *except*:

A. Photosensitivity rash

B. Unexplained proteinuria

C. Thrombocytopenia

D. False-positive testing for syphilis

E. Multiple spontaneous abortions

C The correct answer is choice **C**—thrombocytopenia. The other answers reflect symptoms or findings manifested frequently in a typical SLE patient. In addition, pleurisy, malaise, and the presence of an intermittent low-grade fever have been reported as other symptoms that should raise a suspicion of SLE. Diagnostic laboratory testing often includes the following: Positive antinuclear antibody test results (greater than 1 in 160), elevated anti-Ro or anti-La antibody titers, decreased C3 or C4 complement levels, a positive lupus anticoagulant test result, and elevated anticardiolipin antibody or anti-double-stranded DNA antibody titers. Thrombocytopenia, however, occurs in approximately 5–7% of all pregnancies. Although it may be associated with a lupus flare, thrombocytopenia is not a pathognomonic finding of SLE. Most commonly, thrombocytopenia results from benign gestational thrombocytopenia. Occasionally, it manifests as part of the HELLP syndrome or secondary to idiopathic thrombocytopenic purpura.

4 Which of the following statements regarding the treatment of SLE in pregnancy is *incorrect*?

A. Corticosteroids are effective agents when used during a lupus flare; side effects include glucose intolerance and hypertension.

B. Antimalarial agents such as hydrochloroquine are strictly contraindicated.

C. Patients suffering from the antiphospholipid-antibody syndrome should use low-dose aspirin and moderate-dose heparin for improved fetal outcome.

D. Safe antihypertensive agents in pregnancy include methyldopa, hydralazine, and labetolol.

B Pharmacologic treatment of SLE during pregnancy involves the familiar calculation of fetal risk versus maternal benefit. Acetaminophen, widely used and well studied, should be the preferred agent for patients contending with only mild musculoskeletal complaints. Women enduring a lupus flare during pregnancy may require oral prednisone therapy. Such patients must be monitored closely for glucose intolerance and gestational diabetes. Moreover, women taking oral steroids during pregnancy for SLE or other processes should, subsequently, use an oral taper. Stress-dose steroid therapy during labor and delivery (i.e., 100 mg hydrocortisone IV every 8 hours) may be indicated as well. Finally, corticosteroid therapy has been independently associated with the development of hypertension. Antihypertensive agents—both oral and parenteral—that are safe in pregnancy include methyldopa, hydralazine, and labetolol. Choices **A**, **C** and **D** are correct statements. Pregnant women who test positive for antiphospholipid antibodies should receive low-dose aspirin and adjusted-dose heparin prophylaxis. A suggested goal is the maintenance of the aPTT ratio at least 1.5 times the control level. Extended use of heparin, however, mandates the surveillance of platelet counts to rule out heparin-induced thrombocytopenia. Twice-daily dosing of a low-molecular-weight heparin such as enoxaparin may be used as a substitute for intravenous heparin. Periodic monitoring of the anti-factor Xa is warranted in patients using enoxaparin.

Choice **B** is incorrect. Some authorities recommend avoiding chloroquine during pregnancy. It is important to note, however, that studies have not shown any adverse effects to the fetus. Moreover, control of SLE with antimalarial agents is preferred to losing control of the disease process during pregnancy.

For Questions 5 and 6, please refer to the following vignette.
A 34-year-old gravida 2 para 1001 presents late in her pregnancy for her first prenatal visit. An ultrasound performed earlier that day corroborates the dating by her last menstrual period; she is 31 weeks pregnant. Her medical history is unremarkable with the exception of chronic hypertension, for which she has never taken any medication. Her office blood pressure is 135/85 and her urine dipstick reveals +1 proteinuria. Laboratory values from that day are within normal limits, save for a markedly elevated aspartate aminotransferase (AST). Physical examination of the patient reveals a nontender and nondistended abdomen.

---

5 The differential diagnosis includes all of the following *except*:

A. HELLP syndrome

B. Viral hepatitis

C. Budd-Chiari syndrome

D. Wilson's disease

E. Acute fatty liver of pregnancy (AFLP)

F. Thrombotic thrombocytopenia purpura (TTP)

C For answer, see the answer to Question 6.

6 All of the following statements regarding acute fatty liver of pregnancy (AFLP) are true *except*:

A. Postpartum liver transplantation should be considered in severe cases.

B. Its serum profile readily distinguishes AFLP from the HELLP syndrome.

C. Poor prognostic indicators include coincident renal impairment, metabolic acidosis, hypotension, and hyponatremia.

D. It is a highly morbid condition.

E. It can often be distinguished from the HELLP syndrome by the presence of profound hypoglycemia.

B Acute fatty liver of pregnancy (AFLP) is an uncommon, albeit devastating, clinical entity with an estimated occurrence rate of 1 in 10,000 deliveries. Despite improved management and inclusion of milder cases, maternal and fetal mortalities still reach approximately 25%. AFLP is often associated with preeclampsia, multiple gestation, and a male fetus. Severe cases often manifest pronounced hypoglycemia, hepatic and renal failure, metabolic acidosis, bleeding diatheses, coma, and death. Laboratory findings confirm hypoglycemia and leukocytosis with a left shift. Other characteristic laboratory findings in AFLP parallel those of the HELLP syndrome: both entities evince elevated liver enzymes and hyperuricemia. Maternal and fetal outcomes do not correlate, however, with AST levels.

Antepartum management of AFLP includes the familiar principles dictating management of the HELLP syndrome: referral to a tertiary center, treatment of any associated hypertension, magnesium sulfate therapy if warranted, close monitoring of signs and symptoms heralding acute hepatic failure, and response to the sequelae of hepatic and renal failure. Postpartum liver transplantation for severe AFLP should be considered.

The correct answer to question 5 is choice **C**. Budd-Chiari syndrome—a venoocclusive disease predisposed by the hypercoagulable state of pregnancy—manifests with abrupt-onset ascites and hepatomegaly with consequent abdominal tenderness and pain. Additionally, AST elevations in Budd-Chiari patients tend to be modest. A markedly elevated AST, however, is plausible in all the other suggested clinical entities. This rather broad differential diagnosis can be narrowed. Hypoglycemia suggests AFLP. Thrombocytopenia raises clinical suspicion for the HELLP syndrome. Kayser-Fleischer rings by slit-lamp analysis suggest Wilson's disease. Schistocytes on a peripheral blood smear points to thrombotic TTP. Appropriate serology can concretize a putative diagnosis of viral hepatitis.

The correct answer to question 6 is choice **B**. As stated above, the serum profile of AFLP does not allow convenient differentiation from the HELLP syndrome.

7 A 25-year-old nulliparous woman seeks preconception counseling from her obstetrician. Her past medical history includes a 5-year history of inflammatory bowel disease (IBD). Which of the following statements is *incorrect?*

A. Ulcerative colitis has not been associated with reduced fertility.

B. Active Crohn's disease during pregnancy predisposes toward premature delivery and low birthweight.

C. Methotrexate therapy for IBD is contraindicated during pregnancy.

D. Women with IBD who conceive should be switched from sulfasalazine to immunomodulator therapy with azathioprine or 6-mercaptopurine.

E. Patients with Crohn's disease with significant perianal scarring should be offered a cesarean delivery.

D The clinical entities that comprise IBD—ulcerative colitis and Crohn's disease—have peak incidence rates among women in their prime child-bearing years, ages 15–35. Hence, IBD and pregnancy often coincide. Ulcerative colitis does not cause impaired fertility. Studies on the effect of Crohn's disease on fertility have yielded conflicting results. Indeed, infertility probably correlates with the degree of disease activity; the presence of pelvic adhesions or inflammation would impair fertility. Patients with active Crohn's disease who do conceive face increased risks of preterm and low-birthweight neonates. Choices **A** and **B** are correct.

Perineal scarring, if sufficiently severe, complicates vaginal delivery, precludes proper healing of a perineal laceration, and poses as a contraindication to episiotomy. Such scarring is far likelier to occur in Crohn's disease than in ulcerative colitis. In this event, a cesarean section may be indicated. Choice **E** is correct as well.

The pharmacologic armamentarium for treatment of IBD includes corticosteroids, sulfasalazine, and immunosuppressive agents including azathioprine, 6-mercaptopurine, cyclosporine, and methotrexate. Sulfasalazine contains 5-amino salicylate, which is inactivated by its coupling to sulfapyridine. Colonic bacteria degrade this bond, thereby releasing the antiinflammatory effect of the salicylate in the colon. Sulfasalazine is considered safe in pregnancy. The hypothetical concern that it may cause kernicterus has not been substantiated in studies. Methotrexate, in contrast, is contraindicated for use during pregnancy (choice **C**). It is an abortifacient with teratogenic activity as well. Immunosuppressive agents such as azathioprine have also been shown to be reasonably safe in pregnancy. Their track record is limited, however. Two options exist for pregnant patients contending with IBD managed by azathioprine. These patients may continue their azathioprine regimen if it has proven effective for them. Alternatively, they can be switched to sulfasalazine—whose safety in pregnancy has been better established—around the time of conception. Choice **D**—implying that azathioprine is a safer and more effective drug—is incorrect. Folate supplementation should accompany sulfasalazine use in pregnancy.

8 A 33-year-old multigravida presents to her obstetrician at 31 weeks' gestation with recent-onset pruritis that is both generalized and severe. On laboratory evaluation, she displays elevated serum total bile acid concentrations, elevated serum aminotransferases, and elevated alkaline phosphatase. Which of the following statements is *correct*?

A. The patient must receive a comprehensive work-up to exclude the HELLP syndrome

B. Patients presenting with this clinical entity face significant hepatic sequelae.

C. Treatment with ursodeoxycholic acid (UDCA) has been demonstrated to ameliorate pruritis, but it neither reverses hepatic laboratory abnormalities nor is it safe for use in pregnancy.

D. Cesarean section is indicated for patients presenting with this condition.

E. Risks to the fetus incurred by this clinical entity include fetal distress with meconium-stained amniotic fluid, preterm delivery, and intrauterine fetal death.

E Intrahepatic cholestasis of pregnancy (ICP), a second- and third-trimester clinical entity, occurs with an incidence rate of 0.2–4%. Genetic factors and increased serum estrogen levels have been implicated in the pathogenesis of ICP. Generalized pruritis functions as both the clinical hallmark of ICP and as an important finding that easily distinguishes ICP from the HELLP syndrome. The characteristic laboratory abnormality is the significantly increased serum total bile acid concentration, with an elevated cholic/chenodeoxycholic acid ratio. Additionally, total bilirubin, aminotransferase, and alkaline phosphatase levels show significant elevation above normal levels. Currently, the best agent used to treat ICP is the synthetic bile acid ursodeoxycholic acid (UDCA). Safely used in pregnancy, UDCA ameliorates pruritis and stabilizes the deranged hepatic laboratory values associated with ICP. For refractory cases of ICP, early delivery may be indicated. The route of delivery, however, should follow routine obstetric considerations. Answer choices **A**, **C**, and **D** are incorrect.

Long-term maternal effects of ICP are inconsequential. Although the recurrence rate reaches 60–70%, affected patients do not typically manifest any hepatic sequelae. Choice **B** is incorrect. Risks to the fetus, however, are of considerable clinical concern. Listed accurately in the selected answer, choice **E**, the risks of fetal distress and intrauterine death motivate some authorities to recommend routine antenatal testing for patients afflicted with ICP.

9 A patient presents to the triage section of a Labor and Delivery suite at 15 weeks' gestation. She complains of right-flank pain, frequent urination with urgency, and a 2-day history of vomiting. Her temperature is 38.6°C. Proper management includes all of the following *except*:

A. Empiric treatment with oral trimethoprim/sulfamethoxazole or nitrofurantoin and careful outpatient monitoring

B. Antibiotic treatment course followed by suppressive therapy with 250 mg ampicillin daily or 100 mg nitrofurantoin daily for the duration of the pregnancy

C. Aggressive intravenous fluid hydration

D. Hospitalization and intravenous administration of cefazolin sodium pending urine culture speciation and sensitivity results

E. Close attention to the risk of subsequent preterm labor or preterm rupture of membranes

A Asymptomatic bacteruria (ASB) associates with preterm delivery and low birthweight. ASB occurs in 2–7% of pregnancies. Untreated, ASB may progress to pyelonephritis in approximately one-quarter of pregnant women. Far more daunting than cystitis, pyelonephritis increases the risk of preterm labor and preterm rupture of membranes. Other complications include bacteremia, sepsis, adult respiratory distress syndrome, and hemolytic anemia. Management, accordingly, entails hospitalization, aggressive intravenous fluid hydration (choice **C**), antipyretic treatment, and intravenous antibiotic therapy. Given the risks of preterm labor and/or rupture of membranes (choice **E**), outpatient management with oral antibiotics should not be attempted. Choice **A** is the selected answer. Cefazolin sodium (Ancef), a first-generation cephalosporin, offers adequate coverage for the overwhelming majority of pregnant patients with pyelonephritis. Pending speciation and sensitivity results from the urine culture, cefazolin should be used (choice **D**). Alternatively, many practitioners treat pyelonephritis during pregnancy empirically, with intravenous ampicillin (clindamycin for the penicillin-allergic patient) plus an aminoglycoside such as gentamicin, and subsequently adjust the regimen according to urine culture results. Intravenous antibiotics should be administered until the patient is afebrile for at least 48 hours. Oral antibiotics may then be substituted for the duration of the 14-day course of treatment. Oral antibiotic regimens include ampicillin, cephalexin (Keflex), nitofurantoin (Macrobid), or trimethoprim/sulfamethoxazole (Bactrim). Fluoroquinolones such as ciprofloxacin are, contraindicated in pregnancy. The recurrence rate of pyelonephritis in pregnancy is 20%. Suppressive therapy—using any of the aforementioned oral antibiotic regimens at one-half the treatment dose—is recommended for the duration of any pregnancy complicated by pyelonephritis (choice **B**).

10 An unregistered patient presents to Labor and Delivery claiming she is at 11 weeks' gestation by her last menstrual period. She had a positive pregnancy test at home soon after missing her period. She complains of a 2-week history of severe nausea and vomiting. Proper management of this patient might entail all of the following *except*:

A. Transabdominal ultrasound to confirm a viable intrauterine pregnancy

B. Intravenous fluids and antiemetic therapy

C. Treatment with pyridoxine

D. Treatment with levothyroxine (synthroid)

E. Thiamine supplementation

D Hyperemesis gravidarum entails severe and refractory nausea and vomiting associated with dehydration, ketonuria, and electrolyte derangement. This entity—most commonly between the eighth and twelfth week of gestation—complicates up to 1% of pregnancies. Treatment entails intravenous fluid resuscitation, antiemetic therapy, and correction of electrolyte disturbances. Thiamine supplementation is advised in severe cases of hyperemesis to avoid Wernicke's encephalopathy. Although the U.S. Food and Drug Administration (FDA) has not specifically approved any drug for the treatment of nausea and vomiting in pregnancy, several agents have been used successfully. They include pyridoxine (vitamin B_6), promethazine (Phenergan), metoclopramide (Reglan), ondansetron (Zofran), and methylprednisolone (Medrol) followed by an appropriate taper. Initial workup for hyperemesis includes a metabolic panel to screen for electrolyte abnormalities, confirmation of a viable intrauterine pregnancy, and thyroid function tests. The latter tests enable exclusion of molar pregnancy, and hyperthyroidism, two clinical entities that commonly cause hyperemesis. Synthroid therapy is therefore inappropriate, and choice **D** is the correct response.

17

Hematologic Disease in Pregnancy

Melissa Yates
Cynthia Holcroft

1 A 19-year-old African-American primigravida at 16-2/7 weeks' gestation presents for an initial obstetric visit. Her registration labs are significant for a hematocrit of 35.6%, Hgb electrophoresis HbAS, with a normal peripheral smear. What test would be important to follow throughout the pregnancy?

A. Nonstress test starting at 32 weeks' gestation
B. Urine culture and sensitivity each trimester
C. Hematocrit every 4 weeks
D. MCV at 28 weeks' gestation
E. Serial growth ultrasound every 3 weeks starting at 24 weeks' gestation

B Women with sickle cell trait are at increased risk of renal infection and should be screened every trimester for urinary tract infections. There is no direct fetal compromise from maternal sickle trait, but the father of the baby should be screened with hemoglobin electrophoresis and MCV to determine the likelihood of the fetus having sickle cell disease (HgbSS, HgbSC, and sickle thalessemia).

2 A 32-year-old Caucasian primigravida delivered an infant with severe thrombocytopenia at 39-5/7 weeks' gestation. The patient had a normal platelet count throughout the pregnancy and had no history of any prior hematologic disorder. The patient most likely had which of the following disorders?

A. Gestational thrombocytopenia
B. HELLP syndrome
C. Idiopathic thrombocytopenic purpura (ITP)
D. Alloimmune thrombocytopenia
E. Thrombotic thrombocytopenic purpura (TTP)

D In alloimmune thrombocytopenia, the mother makes antibodies against a paternal antigen on the fetal platelets. This disease is essentially the platelet equivalent of hemolytic (Rh) disease of the newborn except that alloimmune thrombocytopenia can occur in the first pregnancy. These antiplatelet antibodies can then cross the placenta into the fetal circulation and cause fetal thrombocytopenia, which may only be diagnosed at delivery in an otherwise normal pregnancy with normal maternal platelet counts. Approximately 10–20% of infants born with this disorder may have intracranial hemorrhage, of which 25–50% occurs *in utero*. These hemorrhages can be manifested on ultrasound as porencephalic cysts and obstructive hydrocephalus.

3 The patient in Question 2 presents 1 year later with a second pregnancy. The mother is found to have antibodies against HPA-1a. The father is noted to be homozygous for HPA-1a. How should testing proceed during this pregnancy?

A. The couple should be offered a genetic termination of pregnancy.
B. Fetal blood sampling should be obtained at 20–22 weeks' gestation.
C. The mother should have platelet counts performed every 4 weeks.
D. The mother should receive a platelet transfusion at delivery.
E. No antepartum management is necessary, because there is no increased risk of recurrence in a second pregnancy.

B There are at least 10 recognized platelet specific antigens noted at this time. The most common in Caucasian patients is HPA-1a. This is the antigen reported more than 50% of the time in alloimmune thrombocytopenia and is noted to be the most severe. The fact that the father is homozygous for this antigen indicates that this next fetus is at risk to have an equally severe or worse disease than the first infant born to this couple. Fetal blood sampling is initiated at 20–22 weeks to determine the initial fetal platelet levels. It is also important to follow the pregnancy with serial sonograms to assess for growth, hydrops, and intracranial hemorrhage. Therapies currently in use include the administration of maternal steroids, maternal administration of IVIG, and/or fetal platelet transfusion using washed, irradiated platelets. Depending on the initial fetal platelet count, fetal blood sampling with fetal platelet and/or blood transfusion may need to be repeated throughout the pregnancy. This procedure can be performed shortly before delivery to assess the most appropriate mode (vaginal versus cesarean section).

4 A 35-year-old primigravida has been on low-molecular-weight heparin (LMWH) anticoagulation twice daily throughout the pregnancy, secondary to a history of homozygous factor V Leiden mutation. Her dose has been deemed therapeutic by serial anti-factor Xa levels. Her pregnancy has been uneventful for any thromboembolic event. The patient is now at 28 weeks' gestation and has been contracting regularly for 18 hours. She discontinued her LMWH injections when she first felt contractions. How long will she have to wait before being able to receive epidural anesthesia safely?

A. 6 hours after the last dose

B. 10–12 hours after the last dose

C. 24 hours after the last dose

D. 72 hours after the last dose

E. 1 week after the last dose

C Patients should stop LMWH at the onset of labor. If the patient were on once-daily dosing, an epidural could be given 10–12 hours after the last dose; for a patient on twice-daily dosing, an epidural should not be given until 24 hours after the last dose.

5 A 23-year-old primigravida was noted to have thrombocytopenia with a platelet count of 10,000 at 16 weeks' gestation. She was asymptomatic and has been treated intermittently with oral steroids throughout the pregnancy, with good response. She is currently at 38 weeks' gestation and presented to Labor and Delivery in labor. Currently her platelet count is 50,000. What intrapartum testing and/or treatment should be offered to the patient before attempting vaginal delivery?

A. Cordocentesis

B. Fetal scalp sampling

C. Maternal platelet antibody level

D. Maternal IVIG

E. No additional treatment and/or testing would be beneficial

E This patient has immune thrombocytopenic purpura. Maternal thrombocytopenia, antiplatelet antibodies, and maternal response to treatment all correlate poorly with neonatal thrombocytopenia. In addition, with ITP, the fetal platelet count reaches its nadir 48–72 hours after birth. Although the neonate is at increased risk of intracranial hemorrhage after delivery, at this time, mode of delivery in patients with ITP is not thought to influence outcome.

18

Alloimmunization

Julie Jolin

1 A 30-year-old gravida 3, para 2, who had two prior uncomplicated pregnancies registers for prenatal care at 10 weeks' gestation. Her initial lab results show that her blood group is B, Rh-negative, with a negative antibody screen. At 28 weeks' gestation, her antibody screen is positive. She confirms to you that her Rh-positive husband is definitely the father of all three pregnancies and that she received Rh immune globulin (RhIg) both antepartum and postpartum with her two past pregnancies. The most important next step in managing this patient is to

A. Administer 300 μg RhIg immediately.

B. Quantify the level of fetomaternal hemorrhage and then administer the appropriate amount of RhIg.

C. Determine the antibody titer and consider amniocentesis if the titer of anti-D is 1:32 or greater.

D. Await delivery and, if the neonate is Rh-negative, do not administer RhIg.

C Management of pregnancy in unsensitized Rh-negative women requires following antibody screens during and after gestation. Initial screening at less than 20 weeks' gestation involves determination of ABa blood group, Rh type, and antibody screen. At 28 weeks' gestation, the antibody screen should be repeated, at which point 300 μg of RhIg should be administered if the results are negative. In this case, the antibody screen results were positive, thus necessitating a change to managing her as an Rh-immunized woman, and obviating the need for RhIg.

Rh-alloimmunized women should be followed closely by titers. Any patient with an anti-D antibody titer higher than 1:4 should be considered Rh-sensitized. Antibody titers higher than 1:16 are generally considered critical titers, requiring further evaluation with amniocentesis beginning at 26 weeks' gestation or earlier. If the antibody titer is less than the critical titer in the first pregnancy of a sensitized woman, titer determination should be repeated every 2–4 weeks, beginning at 16–18 weeks' gestation. Current management also includes fetal middle cerebral artery Doppler velocimetry to estimate the degree of fetal anemia.

2 A 24-year-old woman, gravida 2, para 1, is being evaluated for delivery at 32 weeks' gestation due to pregnancy affected by Rh sensitization. Her first pregnancy was complicated by intrauterine transfusion, early delivery, and neonatal exchange transfusion. In this pregnancy, gestational dates were confirmed by an 8-week ultrasound, and the father, who is Rh-positive, is confirmed to be the only possible father. Serial ultrasounds in this pregnancy have revealed no evidence of hydrops. Amniocentesis starting at 26 weeks' gestation revealed optical densities in Liley zone I or lower zone II, until the latest amniocentesis, which fell into the upper zone II of the Liley graph. Important next steps in the management of this patient include:

A. Continue to follow the patient with amniocentesis every 2–4 weeks, with further intervention if the optical density reaches Liley zone III.

B. Repeat amniocentesis in 7–14 days, perform cordocentesis if the optical density trends upward, and provide intrauterine transfusion for hematocrit < 30%.

C. Repeat amniocentesis in 7–14 days and perform cordocentesis if the optical density trends downward.

D. Immediate delivery regardless of fetal lung maturity.

B In pregnancies complicated by Rh sensitization, performing a first amniocentesis depends on obstetric history, maternal titers, and gestational age. Subsequent management is based on the amniotic fluid and where it falls on an optical density zones graph, named for its originator, Liley. Since Liley's description in the 1960s, spectrophotometric examination of amniotic fluid has allowed quantification of bilirubin concentrations, which has been shown to correlate with severity of fetal hemolysis in cases of Rh sensitization. Obstetric management is based specifically on Liley values: a repeat amniocentesis is recommended in 2–4 weeks for densities in Liley zone I or lower zone II, with delivery when lung maturity is present. A repeat amniocentesis in 7–10 days is recommended for densities in middle or upper Liley zone II. Then, if the values trend downward, another repeat amniocentesis in 7–14 days is appropriate, while a cordocentesis with possible intrauterine transfusion based on levels of anemia is necessary if the values trend flat or upward. Finally, for Liley zone III, delivery is recommended for gestations greater than 32–34 weeks' gestation with fetal lung maturity present, but cordocentesis with possible transfusion is an option for those with absent lung maturity. In addition to assessment of amniotic fluid bilirubin or umbilical cord hematocrit, daily monitoring of fetal movements by patients after 26–28 weeks' gestation, nonstress tests one to two times weekly, and ultrasonographic examinations every 1–2 weeks are recommended.

19

Surgical Disease in Pregnancy

Francisco Rojas

1 A 22-year-old woman, gravida 1 para 0, presents at 30 weeks' gestation to the emergency room with a 12-hour history of abdominal pain, followed by mild fever, one episode of vomiting, and recent anorexia. Her vital signs are temperature of 101.5°F (38.7°C), blood pressure 120/75, pulse 104, and physical exam is remarkable for voluntary guarding on palpation of the right flank, but no masses or tenderness on the right lower abdominal quadrant. Rebound is not present. Bowel sounds are diminished but present. Fetal heart rate is 156 beats per minute. White blood cell count is 15,500 with 5% bands. The patient is in the left lateral decubitus position and receiving supplemental oxygen. External fetal heart rate monitoring is reassuring. Your next step in managing this condition is

A. Reevaluate in 12–18 hours
B. Start tocolytic agents
C. Open laparoscopy
D. Laparotomy
E. Start antibiotics

D Acute appendicitis is the most common surgical complication of pregnancy (1 in 1,500 pregnancies). However, the classical presentation of appendicitis is usually distorted in the presence of pregnancy, and a high clinical suspicion is essential in order to make an early diagnosis. If the delay in diagnosis is longer than

24 hours, maternal mortality may approach 5%. The role of tocolytic agents perioperatively is not known. Laparoscopy is contraindicated during the third trimester of pregnancy. Antibiotics should be administrated in cases of perforation, abscess, or peritonitis. The acceptable rate of laparotomy with negative findings is 20–35% under these circumstances.

2 An alcohol-related motor vehicle accident (MVA) involved a 28-year-old gravida 2, para 1001, at 34 weeks' gestation, who arrives to the emergency department with Glasgow coma scale of 10, blood pressure 70/40, pulse 112, temperature 98.5°F, oxygen saturation 98% on room air. Lungs are clear bilaterally. A nonopen fracture is evident in the left femur. Cervical spotting is noted during pelvic exam. Fetal heart rate is 120 beats per minute. The most appropriate next step is

A. Oxygen by nasal cannula
B. Kleithauer-Betke test
C. Stabilization of the mother
D. Fracture reduction
E. Cesarean section

C One in 12 pregnancies is complicated by trauma. MVA is the most common cause. Even though this patient has a high risk for a complicated femur fracture with secondary massive bleeding or placental abruption, the mother should first be stabilized. Airway, breathing, and circulation must be established and maintained with the same criteria as in nonpregnant patients. This rule is especially important in patients with altered sensorium and unexplained shock. Frequently, nonreassuring fetal heart status will improve with maternal stabilization. If not, it may be managed when the mother is stable.

3 A 19-year-old primigravida at 22 weeks' gestation was injured with a shotgun 15 minutes ago. Upon arrival to the emergency room, her vitals signs are temperature 98.9°F, blood pressure 115/75, pulse 100, respiratory rate 22. She is oriented, alert, and coherent, with normal heart sounds and clear lungs bilaterally. Her abdomen shows only an entrance wound on her left flank, without guarding, without rebound, present bowel sounds. Her cervix is closed and long, without bleeding or leaking of amniotic fluid. Fetal heart rate is 136 beats per minute. The next step in her treatment is

A. Tetanus toxoid
B. CBC, type and screen, cross match
C. Local exploration of the wound
D. Peritoneal lavage
E. Laparotomy

E Management of pregnant patients with penetrating trauma is the same as that of nonpregnant women. Surgical exploration is mandatory in gunshot wounds to the abdomen or flank. Tetanus toxoid, CBC, type and screen, and cross match are useful but cannot replace laparotomy in this clinical scenario. Local exploration of the wound and peritoneal lavage are not appropriate for gunshot wounds.

20

Postpartum Care and Breastfeeding

Julia Cron

1 In treating endomyometritis, ampicillin is added to cover which of the following organisms?

A. *Staphylococcus*

B. *Enterococcus*

C. *Pseudomonas*

D. *Trichomonas*

B Ampiciliin is added to increase the synergistic effects of treatment on *Enterococcus faecalis*.

2 A 29-year-old gravida 1, para 1, has just had a vaginal delivery after pitocin induction for severe preeclampsia. Her induction began 21 hours ago. After delivery, you inspect the perineum, vagina, and cervix, and find no lacerations or tears. The patient then begins to have heavy vaginal bleeding. What is the best immediate intervention?

A. Check coagulation factors

B. Bolus pitocin

C. Uterine massage

D. McCall's stitch

E. Cesarean hysterectomy

C The most likely etiology is uterine atony secondary to prolonged pitocin induction, although in the setting of severe preeclampisa, a coagulopathy should always be considered. The first management approach should be vigorous uterine massage. If uterotonic agents are required, pitocin followed by a prostaglandin agonist should be administered. Ergot derivatives are contraindicated in the setting of preeclampsia or hypertension.

3 A 32-year-old gravida 3, para 2012, presents for routine medical care 1 year after the birth of her child. She had gestational diabetes with both of her pregnancies. She is mildly obese and has no other medical problems. Her mother has end-stage disease secondary to diabetes. She has no medical complaints. You would like to screen her for diabetes, so you obtain a fasting glucose, which is 140 mg/dL. How should you proceed?

A. Obtain another level after 2 hours

B. Obtain another fasting glucose another day

C. Perform an adrenal challenge test with a glucose load

D. Begin therapy with a daily oral hypoglycemic if she becomes symptomatic

E. Refer to an endocrinologist

B Given her history of gestational diabetes, her obesity, and her family history of diabetes, it is appropriate to screen this patient annually for nongestational diabetes. Her fasting glucose level is abnormal, but the diagnosis of diabetes requires confirmation of an abnormal value on a different day. You could obtain another fasting glucose (normal < 100 mg/dL, carbohydrate-intolerant 110–125 mg/dL, diabetes 2 type 126 mg/dL) or check a glucose level 2 hours after a 75-g load (normal < 140 mg/dL, carbohydrate-intolerant 140–199 mg/dL, diabetes type 2, 200 mg/dL).

4 Which of the following women would be counseled *against* breastfeeding?

A. A woman with HIV in an isolated rural village in a less developed country

B. A woman who just delivered, at term, an otherwise healthy baby with cytomegalovirus (CMV)

C. A woman with active, untreated tuberculosis

D. A woman with chronic hepatitis B with no evidence of active liver disease, whose infant received hepatitis B immunoglobulin and the hepatitis B vaccine

E. All of the above

C HIV is found in breast milk and thus, in the developed world, where infant formula is readily available, women with HIV are encouraged against breastfeeding. However, in underdeveloped countries, where infant malnutrition is a major cause of infant mortality, breastfeeding is encouraged in most circumstances, including maternal HIV infection. Infants born to mothers with tuberculosis may receive expressed breast milk once the treatment regimen is well established.

5 A 25-year-old gravida 3, para 2012, presents 4 weeks postpartum with concerns about a breast mass. She had been seen 1 week ago with complaints of fever and erythema of the right breast. She was started on dicloxacillin for presumed mastitis. On physical exam today, you note a temperature of 38.3°C and a firm, 2 × 2 cm, extremely tender mass in the left lower quadrant of the right breast. How do you proceed?

A. Start intravenous antibiotics

B. Obtain ultrasound of breast

C. Immediate incision and drainage

D. Refer to breast surgeon

B A breast abscess is a complication that may result from mastitis. Ultrasound is required for diagnosis. If confirmed by ultrasonography, treatment is incision and drainage.

21

Obstetric Analgesia and Anesthesia

Betty Chou

1 A 36-year-old gravida 2, para 1, at 39-4/7 weeks' gestation presents to Labor and Delivery in active labor. Her cervix is 4 cm dilated and 100% effaced, and the fetal head is at −1 station. After receiving an epidural for anesthesia, an amniotomy is performed to expedite the progression of labor. Thirty minutes later, repetitive mild late decelerations are noted on the fetal heart tracing. The patient's blood pressure is noted to be 82/40. On exam, the patient's cervix is 5 cm dilated and there is no evidence of vaginal bleeding or cord prolapse. Maternal hypotension secondary to epidural anesthesia is believed to be the cause of the late decelerations of the fetal heart rate. After the patient is placed into the left lateral tilt position and 1 L of intravenous fluid is administered, the fetal late decelerations persist. What is the next best intervention?

A. Prompt cesarean section

B. Scalp pH

C. Repeat intravenous saline fluid boluses

D. Intravenous ephedrine administration

D Epidural anesthesia is generally a very safe and effective mode of analgesia and anesthesia for the laboring obstetric patient. However, there are risks associated. The most common risk is maternal hypotension, which can cause uteroplacental insufficiency and fetal distress. Before an epidural is placed, the patient should receive an intravenous fluid bolus as a prophylaxis against maternal hypotension. If maternal hypotension still occurs, the first steps of treatment are left lateral tilt positioning and an additional intravenous fluid bolus. If these interventions do not resolve the maternal hypotension and fetal distress persists, the next best step is to administer intravenous ephedrine, which increases maternal systemic blood pressure and blood return to the placenta. Other causes of fetal distress must be excluded before assuming that maternal hypotension secondary to epidural is the etiology. For example, in the above case, abruption and cord prolapse were considered before giving ephedrine.

Neither prompt cesarean section nor scalp pH is the next best intervention in this case. If ephedrine is administered and the nonreassuring fetal heart rate pattern resolves, the patient is spared from having a scalp pH or urgent surgery. However, if ephedrine is administered and the maternal blood pressure normalizes while the fetal heart tracing continues to show late decelerations, further interventions may be warranted.

2 An 18-year-old gravida 1, para 0, at 40-2/7 weeks' gestation presents to Labor and Delivery complaining of contractions and leakage of fluid for the last 5 hours. On exam, the patient is found to have grossly ruptured fetal membranes, leaking clear fluid. Her cervix is 7 cm dilated, 100% effaced, and the presenting part is at 0 station. Exam and sonography demonstrate that the fetus is in the double-footling breech position. The patient has no medical problems and her laboratory studies are unremarkable. The decision is made to proceed with a cesarean section. What is the best mode of anesthesia?

A. General anesthesia

B. Spinal anesthesia

C. Epidural anesthesia

D. Local anesthesia

B Spinal anesthesia is ideal for this situation specifically, because of the rapid onset of effect and ease of administration. The patient is already 7 cm dilated and may progress quickly in labor. She does not have the time that may be required to administer and dose an epidural.

In addition, the patient does not have any contraindications to spinal anesthesia, such as neurologic or spine abnormalities, infection at the site, acute maternal hemorrhage, or bleeding disorders.

General anesthesia is usually not the anesthetic mode of choice for cesarean delivery unless regional anesthesia is contraindicated. Risks of general anesthesia include failed intubation and aspiration, maternal hypertension, increased uterine bleeding, and fetal depression. In addition, the patient is unconscious and unable to experience the joys associated with delivery.

Local anesthesia is used only in extremely rare emergency occasions for cesarean delivery. Only when a patient needs an emergency cesarean delivery and alternative forms of anesthesia are not immediately available or possible should local anesthesia even be considered. Local anesthesia alone is usually inadequate pain relief.

3 A 39-year-old gravida 5, para 4, at 32-2/7 weeks' gestation presents to Labor and Delivery complaining of painful contractions and heavy vaginal bleeding for the past 3 hours. She is a known cocaine and heroin intravenous drug abuser with a history of hepatitis C and cirrhosis of the liver. On exam, her cervix is found to be 1 cm dilated and long. There is evidence of profuse, bright red vaginal bleeding. Fetal heart tracing shows repetitive mild to moderate late decelerations. A sonogram is performed, which demonstrates a fundal placenta with a large retroplacental clot. Placental abruption is suspected. Laboratory studies are as follows:

- Hct = 20%
- INR = 1.9
- ALT = 250 IU/L
- AST = 300 U/L
- Alb = 2.4 g/dL

The patient requires an emergency cesarean section under general anesthesia. All of the following are indications for general anesthesia in this patient *except*:

A. Urgency of cesarean section

B. Coagulopathy

C. Cirrhosis

D. Hypovolemia

C This patient is having placental abruption, probably secondary to her use of cocaine. The large abruption and profuse blood loss are both causing fetal distress. An emergency cesarean section is necessary. General anesthesia is usually not the anesthetic mode of choice for cesarean deliveries because of increased uterine blood loss, risk of failed intubation, and fetal depression. However, general anesthesia is indicated in patients who need rapid induction for emergency surgery or have contraindications for regional anesthesia. Contraindications to a spinal or epidural include neurologic problems (e.g., sciatica), spinal abnormalities (e.g., severe scoliosis or prior spine fusions), and infection at the site. In addition, acute maternal hemorrhage (causing hypovolemia) and bleeding abnormalities are also contraindications to regional anesthesia.

This patient has several reasons to utilize general anesthesia. With the degree of maternal hemorrhage and fetal distress, the cesarean section is quite emergent. There is also evidence of hypovolemia, as her hematocrit is only 20% and she is still bleeding heavily. Finally, she has bleeding abnormalities with an elevated INR of 1.9. It is unclear whether her coagulopathy is secondary to her cirrhosis or extreme blood loss. Women can have cirrhosis without affecting their bleeding times. Therefore, cirrhosis alone is not a contraindication to regional anesthesia.

22

Anatomy of the Female Pelvis

Courtney Rhoades

1 A 57-year-old thin, postmenopausal woman who is 2 days postoperative from a total abdominal hysterectomy and Burch procedure for uterine prolapse and cystocele is complaining of numbness of her right medial thigh. The patient is able to ambulate, void spontaneously, and pass flatus. She is continent of stool and urine. On exam, she has change of sensation over her right medial thigh but is able to feel sharp and dull sensation. Her reflexes in her extremities are intact. Pulses are intact and she has no swelling in her extremities. Muscle strength is intact except for some weakness of adduction of the right leg. Her sensory motor changes are most likely to represent damage to which nerve?

A. Obturator nerve

B. Perineal nerve

C. Genitofemoral nerve

D. Femoral nerve

E. Femoral cutaneous nerve

A The patient's deficit most likely represents entrapment of the obturator nerve. While retractors can damage the genitofemoral nerve, a solely sensory nerve, as it runs on top of the psoas muscle, the deficit in this patient is sensory and motor. The femoral cutaneous nerve supplies the anterior aspect of the thigh, which is not the deficit presented. The perineal nerve supplies the muscles of the superficial compartment of the vulva. The femoral nerve could be damaged, but the lesion is very specific and injury to the femoral nerve is more likely to cause a motor and sensory defect that would cause difficulty with ambulation. The obturator nerve is easily injured during tumor debulking, lymph node dissection, and a Burch procedure. It can be entrapped at the location of the obturator canal by the sutures. Risk factors include thin body habitus, Pfannenstiel incision, and dorsal lithotomy position.

2 You are performing a total abdominal hysterectomy for an 18-weeks'-size uterus with multiple uterine myomata. Once you have made a Pfannensteil incision and opened the peritoneum, you realize that you require greater exposure to safely complete the surgery. Your next step is to

A. Perform a Maylard incision

B. Convert to a vertical incision

C. Convert to a Cherney incision

C Converting to a Cherney incision (separating the rectus muscles at their tendinous insertion into the symphysis pubis) will give the surgeon better visualization with minimal effect on the patient's postoperative morbidity. A Maylard incision is a transverse incision midway between the pubic bone and umbilicus. The Maylard incision does not involve separating the muscles from the fascia, but does include a transverse incision of both rectus muscles. Closure of the fascia also reapproximates the muscle bodies. Cutting the muscles after a Pfannenstel incision is inappropriate, as the muscles cannot be reapproximated after the rectus muscles have already been dissected off the rectus sheath. Converting to a vertical incision would give better visualization and operating space, but the postoperative morbidity and wound healing would be much worse in a patient with both a vertical and a Pfannesteil incision. Therefore, trying a Cherney incision first would give the patient the chance for less morbidity while affording more room to get around a large uterus.

3 You are performing a laparoscopy on a patient and are about to start removing the trocars at the end of the procedure when you visualize an expanding hematoma forming around the right lower quadrant port. The vessels most likely transected with your trocar are

A. Superficial epigastric artery and vein

B. Deep circumflex iliac artery and vein

C. Inferior epigastric artery and vein

D. Superficial external pudendal artery and vein

E. Superficial circumflex iliac artery and vein

C The inferior epigastric artery and vein run from the external iliac vessels to the umbilicus. They can be seen by laparoscope and form the lateral umbilical fold. They often are sites of hematoma formation secondary to trocar trauma because of their position in the abdomen. The superficial epigastric vessels that lie under the skin in the subcutaneous fatty layer can cause subcuticular hematomas. The superficial external pudendal vessels run from the femoral vessels to the mons pubis and are unlikely to be transected in this case. The superficial circumflex iliac artery and vein run laterally from the femoral vessels and would not be in the area of a lower quadrant trocar. The deep circumflex iliac vessels lie between the internal oblique and transverses abdominus muscles. A hematoma that forms after transection of these vessels is unlikely to be seen by the laparoscope, and port placement is not in close proximity to them.

4 There are six surgical spaces in the pelvis; please match the following:

1. Space of Retzius
2. Rectovaginal space
3. Paravesical space
4. Vesicovaginal and vesicocervical space
5. Pararectal space
6. Retrorectal and presacral space

A. Bordered by ureter and rectum medially and hypogastric vessels laterally

B. Bordered medially by bladder and obliterated umbilical artery, laterally by obturator internus, and dorsally by cardinal ligament

C. Bordered by rectum ventrally, rectal pillars, and uterosacral ligaments laterally, and sacrum dorsally

D. Bordered by cervix, uterosacral ligaments, and rectum

E. Bordered by bladder, vagina, and cervix

F. Bordered by transversalis fascia and rectus muscles, pubocervical ligament, and bladder

Answers:

1. F
2. D
3. B
4. E
5. A
6. C

5 Alcock's canal in the lesser sciatic notch contains which nerve?

A. Pudenal nerve

B. Inferior hemorrhoidal

C. Femoral nerve

D. Genitofemoral nerve

A The pudendal nerve runs from its origin in the sacral plexus through the greater sciatic notch around the ischial spine and then enters Alcock's canal. The inferior hemorrhoidal supplies the external anal sphincter and does not go through the canal. The femoral nerve passes under the inguinal ligament and into the femoral sheath and does not go through the canal. The genitofemoral nerve lies on the psoas muscle and also does not go through the canal of Alcock.

23

Perioperative Care and Complications of Gynecologic Surgery

Eli Rybak

1 Which one of likely following surgical scenarios is associated with the least risk of ureteral injury?

A. Laparoscopic fulguration of endometriosis in a 36-year-old infertility patient

B. Ovarian tumor debulking in a patient with no prior surgical history

C. Extirpation of a tuboovarian abscess (TOA) in a 29-year-old woman

D. Total abdominal hysterectomy (TAH) in a 42-year-old patient with symptomatic uterine leiomyomata

E. Total vaginal hysterectomy in a 40-year-old woman with dysfunctional uterine bleeding

E Although ureteral injury complicates only 0.3–0.5% of cases in gynecologic surgery, nonetheless, the gynecologist must incessantly and vigilantly track the ureter when performing pelvic surgery. Caution is particularly warranted when operating in the presence of a distorted pelvic anatomy. Herein, the ureters are often drawn precariously close to the female reproductive organs. Disorders that increase inflammation, adhesion, formation, or fibrosis in the pelvis greatly facilitate the likelihood of encountering ureteral injury (choices **A** and **C**). Endometriosis, in fact, is the most common diagnosis among patients who sustain ureteral injury from laparoscopy. Mass effect from ovarian malignancy or fibroids likewise potentiate the risk of distorted anatomy and ureteral involvement (choices **B** and **D**). Choice **E**, however, is correct. Of ureteral injuries caused by gynecologic surgery, 75% occur from abdominal procedures and 25% from vaginal procedures. A total vaginal hysterectomy for dysfunctional uterine bleeding is least likely to result in ureteral injury.

2 You are contending with suboptimal visualization while performing a total abdominal hysterectomy and bilateral Salpingo-oophorectomy (TAH-BSO). During the procedure, you suspect an insult to ureteral integrity. Which one of the following statements regarding optimal management in this situation is *correct*?

A. Cystoscopy following the intravenous administration of indigo carmine dye provides for convenient and accurate detection of ureteral injury.

B. Intravenous pyelography (IVP) is 100% sensitive in confirming ureteral injury.

C. Ureteroneocystostomy is the preferred procedure for ureteral injuries proximal to the pelvic brim.

D. Transureteroureterostomy is a first-line procedure for ureteral injuries that are distant from the ureterovesical junction.

E. Stenting the injured ureter is not recommended; stenting promotes iatrogenic injury.

A The gynecologist has several options when he or she suspects ureteral injury. Efflux of the intravenously administered indigo carmine dye within several minutes from each ureteral orifice confirms ureteral patency (choice **A**). Studies reporting the identification of up to 90% of unsuspected ureteral injuries by routine use of cystoscopy warrant its consideration at the conclusion of all major gynecologic surgery. Although intravenous pyelography may be performed intraoperatively as well, it is more cumbersome. More important, small leaks may be missed. The false-negative rate for the detection of ureteral injury by IVP can approach 7%. (choice **B**). Corrective surgical intervention is certainly appropriate in various instances of ureteral injury. Ureteroneocystotomy, however, should only be contemplated for ureteral injuries within approximately 5 cm of the bladder, and not for those proximal to the pelvic brim (choice **C**). Regardless of the location of the ureteral injury, transureteroureterostomy should remain a carefully considered procedure of last resort, secondary to the risks it poses to the functioning ureter (choice **D**). Finally, routine perioperative placement of ureteral stents remains controversial because of the widely shared concern that it promotes iatrogenic injury. Stenting an injured ureter to prevent stricture formation and allow for revascularization, however, is universally mandated (choice **E**).

3 Potential ureteral injury is associated with all of the following steps executed during a TAH *except*:

A. Division of the round ligament

B. Ligation of the infundibulopelvic ligament

C. Ligation of the uterine arteries

D. Clamping of the cardinal ligaments

A A clear knowledge of the path traversed by the ureter as it courses from the pelvic brim to the ureterovesical junction enables the practitioner to identify the common sites of ureteral injury, and to exercise vigilance during the segments of gynecologic surgery occurring at these locations. Upon descending beyond the pelvic brim, the ureter passes anteriorly to the bifurcation of the common iliac artery. As the ureter approaches the ischial spines, it can be located medial to the internal iliac artery and the anterior division branches. Subsequent tracking of the ureter beneath the uterine artery places the ureter only 1.5–2.0 cm lateral to the cervix at the level of the internal os. Finally, the ureter enters the tunnel of the cardinal ligament ("water under the bridge") and passes anteromedially over the vaginal fornix as it enters the trigone region of the bladder.

A gynecologist must, accordingly, exercise caution when operating in one of the five areas predisposed by proximity to ureteral injury. These locations are as follows:

1. Base of the broad ligament
2. Beyond the uterine vessels, as the ureters course medially through the cardinal ligament towards the bladder (choices **C** and **D**)
3. Segment of ureter traversing the bladder wall
4. Region of the infundibulopelvic ligament (choice **B**)
5. Lateral pelvic side wall adjacent to the uterosacral ligament

Choice **A**, division of the round ligament, is ordinarily performed at a safe distance from the ureter.

4 Which statement regarding genitourinary fistulae is *correct*?

A. In the United States, most genitourinary fistulae result from obstetric trauma.

B. When using the tampon test of Moir to detect fistulae, a wet but undyed upper tampon suggests urine loss through the urethra.

C. When using the tampon test, a wet but undyed upper tampon suggests a vesicovaginal fistula.

D. If the tampon test result suggests an ureterovaginal fistula, further appropriate steps include cystoscopy and intravenous pyelography.

E. Fistulae are often detected by the presence of fever, chills, and pelvic pain.

D Although genitourinary (GU) fistulae may present with fever, chills, or pelvic pain (choice **E**), they more commonly present with clear vaginal discharge without any associated constitutional symptoms. The primary cause of GU fistulae in the United States is gynecologic surgery, often a total abdominal hysterectomy performed for benign conditions. Obstetric-related fistulae are less prevalent, as practitioners eschew the difficult forceps delivery and rely increasingly on cesarean section (choice **A**).

The tampon test of Moir is a useful technique to differentiate among a ureterovaginal fistula, vesicovaginal fistula, and urethral incontinence. Methylene blue or indigo carmine dye is applied in retrograde fashion through a Foley transurethral catheter. Three tampons are subsequently placed in the vagina. A wet but undyed upper tampon suggests a ureterovaginal fistula. A wet and blue-dyed upper tampon points to a vesicovaginal fistula. Finally, a wet and blue-dyed bottom tampon implicates urethral incontinence. Choices **B** and **C** are, accordingly, incorrect. Choice **D** is correct; cystoscopy and/or intravenous pyelography are indicated to verify the presence of an ureterovaginal fistula.

5 A 38-year-old patient has a past medical history notable for asthma and a congenital ventricular septal defect (VSD) repaired at birth. She requires albuterol therapy for her asthma, and recently experienced an asthma exacerbation controlled by oral prednisone. Her gynecologic history is remarkable for long-standing diagnoses of infertility and metrorrhagia. She now presents to her gynecologist for operative laparoscopy and hysteroscopy to perform lysis of pelvic adhesions and removal of an endometrial polyp. Proper preoperative management of the patient's asthma and VSD entail:

A. Hydrocortisone, 100 mg IV, at the time of surgery, plus subacute bacterial endocarditis (SBE) prophylaxis with IV ampicillin and gentamicin

B. Preoperative pulmonary function testing and 100 mg methylprednisolone IV at the time of surgery

C. Preoperative albuterol nebulizer treatment and a basic metabolic panel

D. Preoperative albuterol nebulizer treatment and SBE prophylaxis with IV ampicillin

B Preoperative assessment and management of any comorbidity must be comprehensive yet cost-effective, for both the low-risk patient with a benign gynecologic disorder and for the medically complicated, elderly, and/or oncology patient.

The pertinent facts about this particular patient are as follows: She is 38 years old, she suffers from asthma responsive to beta$_2$-agonist and steroid therapy, and she had a congenital ventricular septal defect repaired at birth.

For a medically uncomplicated patient under age 40, a CBC and either a urine or serum pregnancy test are required preoperative tests. Results from a Pap smear obtained within the past 12 months should be available. A basic metabolic panel, ECG, and chest X-ray would not ordinarily be required. In this particular situation, it may be advised to obtain the latter two tests because the patient presents with a cardiac history and reactive airway disease.

Patients contending with asthma who have required oral steroid therapy during the 12-month span preceding their surgery should undergo preoperative pulmonary function testing and stress-dose steroids at the time of surgery. Commonly used 100 mg hydrocortisone IV or 100 mg methylprednisolone IV therapies include (choice **B**). Preoperative nebulizer treatment with albuterol alone is insufficient therapy for this patient (choice **C**). Finally, regarding prophylaxis for subacute bacterial endocarditis, the American Heart Association has revised the recommendations for prophylactic antibiotics administered preoperatively. Patients are now stratified into a high-risk, moderate-risk, or negligible-risk category, and only the former two categories warrant prophylaxis. This patient's cardiac history places her into the negligible-risk category; she does not require preoperative antibiotics (choices **A** and **D**).

6 Which statement regarding vessel injury caused by Veress needle or trocar insertion is *incorrect*?

A. Superficial epigastric vessels can be identified and thus avoided by transillumination in most circumstances.

B. Inferior epigastric vessels can be avoided by inserting the trocars 6 cm lateral to the midline.

C. Elevation of the anterior abdominal wall reduces the risk of injury to blood vessels and internal organs.

D. Significant hemorrhage is managed, in part, by fluid resuscitation with 0.45% normal saline, and transfusion with packed red blood cells, fresh frozen plasma, and platelets in a 2:1:1 ratio.

E. Bleeding can be controlled by cauterization, suture ligation, and tamponade with a Foley catheter balloon.

D Many steps have been shown to reduce the risk of injury to both major and minor blood vessels in the omentum, mesentery, abdomen, and pelvis during insertion of the Veress needle or trocar. These include transillumination (choice **A**), proper lateral placement of the trocars (choice **B**), and elevation of the anterior abdominal wall (choice **C**). The options for managing bleeding listed in choice **E**—cauterization, suture ligation, and tamponade—are correct. Choice **D**, however, is false. Intraoperative hemorrhage mandates every attempt to preserve clear visualization of the affected area, localization of the source of bleeding, and intervention to stop the hemorrhage. If a significant blood loss occurs, hemodynamic stability must be restored by fluid resuscitation and transfusion with blood products. For intravascular volume expansion, normal saline (0.9%) or lactated Ringers solution must be infused. Hypotonic (maintenance) solutions such as one-half-normal saline (0.45%) will not achieve the requisite volume expansion. Finally, blood products are transfused as follows. Each unit of transfused packed red blood cells should elevate the hematocrit by approximately 3%. One unit of fresh frozen plasma is administered for approximately every 4 units of transfused packed red blood cells. If 10 units of packed red blood cells are transfused, 10 units of platelets are administered as well.

7 Which of the following statements regarding fluid monitoring during hysteroscopy is *correct*?

A. 3% Sorbitol is likelier than Hyskon solution to cause volume expansion and pulmonary edema.

B. Excessive administration of hypertonic solutions—such as 1.5% glycine—may trigger arrhythmias and cerebral edema.

C. When sorbitol or mannitol are used for hysteroscopy, a 1,000-mL deficit requires a check of serum sodium level, administration of 20 mg furosemide IV, and termination of the procedure if the serum sodium level falls below 125 mEq/L.

D. When sorbitol or mannitol are used for hysteroscopy, a 2,000-mL deficit requires a check of serum sodium level, administration of 40 mg furosemide IV, and termination of the procedure if the serum sodium level falls below 125 mEq/L.

C Because fluid introduced into the uterine cavity during hysteroscopy may reach the systemic circulation via the endometrial and myometrial blood vessels, the quality and quantity of the fluid being introduced is of critical importance. Hyskon is a 32% solution of dextran 70. The hypertonicity of Hyskon—far exceeding that of 3% sorbitol or 1.5% glycine—threatens precipitous volume expansion and pulmonary edema. Hypotonic solutions, alternatively, trigger a net fluid shift intracellularly. This results in arrhythmias and cerebral edema. Choices **A** and **B** are incorrect.

To prevent the occurrence of uncontrolled fluid shifts during hysteroscopy, various procedures are implemented to accurately calculate both the inflow and outflow of the given fluid. Many management protocols exist regarding further surveillance and/or halting the hysteroscopy procedure if any significant disparity between the calculated inflow and outflow is detected. The management recommendations cited in the *Johns Hopkins Manual of Gynecology and Obstetrics* conform to choice **C**. Unlike the statement in choice **D**, a 2,000-mL fluid deficit actually warrants immediate termination of the procedure. A 1,000-mL deficit merely warrants furosemide therapy and a check of the serum sodium level; the procedure itself, however, may proceed pending a sodium level $\geq$ 125 mEq/L.

8 An obese 58-year-old patient undergoes a prolonged TAH–BSO and endures a complicated postoperative course.

Which of the following statements regarding iatrogenic femoral nerve injury is incorrect?

A. Risk factors include prolonged operating time, the use of a wide Pfannenstiel incision, poorly developed rectus muscles, and a narrow pelvis.

B. Proper positioning of a patient in stirrups minimizes the incidence of intraoperative femoral nerve injury.

C. The use of self-retaining retractors with deep blades minimizes the incidence of intraoperative femoral nerve injury.

D. A patient with postoperative femoral neuropathy often cannot raise her leg straight up while lying in the supine position; a diminished knee-jerk response is common as well.

E. Evidence of a postoperative femoral neuropathy warrants imaging studies to exclude a retroperitoneal hematoma.

C Gynecologic surgery—and particularly, abdominal hysterectomy—is the most frequent cause of iatrogenic femoral nerve injury, with reported incidences exceeding 10%. Emerging from the lateral border of the psoas muscle, the femoral nerve traverses between the psoas and iliacus muscles prior to coursing beneath the inguinal ligament and into the thigh. Motor branches of the femoral nerve innervate the iliac, quadriceps, pectineal, and sartorius muscles; sensory branches innervate the anteromedial aspect of the thigh and leg. Femoral nerve injury results from compression, ligation, transection, or stretch. Risk factors for such injury are numerous, foremost of which is the improper placement of self-retaining retractors (e.g., Balfour or Bookwalter), and especially those outfitted with particularly long or deep blades. Choice **C** is false, and it is the selected answer. The risk factors listed in choice **A** are accurate. A wide Pfannenstiel incision, thin body habitus, poorly developed rectus muscles, and narrow pelvis predispose to femoral nerve injury secondary to a greater likelihood of femoral nerve impingement. Additional cited risk factors include diabetes mellitus, smoking, and general anesthesia. Excessive flexion of the thigh with abduction and external rotation of the hip—a position often exaggerated by the improper positioning of patients in "candy cane" stirrups—predisposes to femoral nerve injury as it exits into the thigh beneath the inguinal ligament. Choice **B** is correct.

Once it is suspected, femoral nerve injury can be confirmed by the characteristic motor—and sensory—deficits associated with femoral neuropathy. Numbness and tingling along the anteromedial aspect of the thigh are complemented by the common motor deficits—specifically, quadriceps weakness—listed correctly in choice **D**. After the diagnosis of femoral nerve injury is confirmed, imaging studies should be obtained to exclude nerve compression secondary to a retroperitoneal hematoma or abscess (choice **E**). Prompt reexploration is indicated if complete transection or suturing of the nerve is suspected. Otherwise, input by a neurologist and physical therapist often facilitate recovery for the majority of patients, whose transient neuropathy can be attributable to retractor or positioning injury.

9 Which of the following statements regarding pulmonary embolus is *incorrect?*

A. Symptoms may include tachypnea, tachycardia, pleuritic chest pain, or hemoptysis.

B. Anticoagulation with a heparin bolus of 80 U/kg IV followed by 18 U/kg per hour is administered until the aPTT ratio is 2.0–2.5.

C. Protamine sulfate reverses heparin-related bleeding.

D. ECG findings of right axis deviation, a Q wave in limb lead III, and an increased pCO_2 obtained from an arterial blood gas confirm the presence of a pulmonary embolus.

E. The spiral chest CT scan is a valid first-line alternative to the ventilation-perfusion (V/Q) scan in the diagnosis of pulmonary embolus.

D Pulmonary embolus (PE) is responsible for 40% of the postoperative mortality among gynecologic patients. Although a PE often presents with its characteristic tachycardia, tachypnea, and respiratory distress, it may occur without initial symptoms. Table 23-8 in the *Johns Hopkins Manual*, Second Edition, refers to the common signs and symptoms associated with PE. Choice **A** accurately lists some of the common symptoms of PE. Choice **B** describes the correct therapeutic dosage for heparin anticoagulation. Choices **A** and **B** are correct. Heparin-related bleeding can be reversed with protamine sulfate (choice **C**); Coumadin-related bleeding can be reversed with vitamin K or fresh frozen plasma. Choice **E** is correct as well: the spiral chest CT scan has, in fact, replaced the ventilation-perfusion scan in many institutions as the fist-line imaging study to rule out PE. Advantages of the CT scan are its speed, accessibility, and reduced susceptibility to interference or confounding by any underlying pulmonary disease. An ambiguous CT scan should be followed up with a ventilation-perfusion scan and, if necessary, by the gold standard, pulmonary angiography.

Choice **D** is incorrect for two reasons. First, PE is associated with tachypnea, hyperventilation, and consequent normal to slightly decreased partial pressure of carbon dioxide on arterial blood gas analysis. Second, ECG findings regarding PE are notoriously nonspecific. Admittedly, PE has been associated with right ventricular strain, right axis deviation, and the "classic" S-wave in limb lead I and both Q-wave and inverted T-wave in limb lead III. These findings serve to heighten one's suspicion of PE; they, alone, do not confirm the diagnosis.

10 Which of the following statements regarding small bowel obstruction (SBO) is *incorrect*?

A. Characteristic abdominal X-ray (AXR) findings include distended loops of small bowel with air–fluid levels.

B. An AXR finding of gas in the colon rules out the presence of a bowel obstruction.

C. Bowel sounds often manifest as high-pitched tinkling sounds.

D. Surveillance of serial white blood cell counts enables the clinician to differentiate between paralytic ileus and advancing bowel obstruction.

E. Risk factors for SBO include adhesions at the operative site, infection, and malignancy.

B Postoperative gastrointestinal (GI) dysfunction often challenges the practitioner to differentiate between an ileus and the potentially more ominous SBO. Both clinical entities share several risk factors, including infection, malignancy, and a history of radiation therapy. Additional risk factors for an ileus include infection, electrolyte derangement, and bowel manipulation. SBO, alternatively, most commonly results from adhesions at the operative site—an occurrence in 1–2% of cases. Choice **E** is, accordingly, true.

Abdominal radiography and clinical assessment of bowel sounds proves helpful—but not always definitive—in differentiating between an ileus and SBO in the distended postoperative patient contending with intractable emesis. AXR findings in cases of SBO reveal distended loops of small bowel, often with air–fluid levels (choice **A**). An ileus may generate similar AXR findings. Often, an ileus can be differentiated from an SBO by the presence of gas in the colon. This finding, however, does not definitively rule out an SBO. Choice **B** is incorrect and is therefore the selected answer. An early or partial SBO may well demonstrate free air in the colon. Indeed, free air in the colon should not alone provide reassurance to the clinician; surveillance of serial white blood cell counts and serial abdominal films are indicated to differentiate between an ileus and a progressing SBO among postoperative patients with persistent GI dysfunction (choice **D**). Finally, an ileus typically manifests absent or hypoactive bowel sounds; high-pitched tinkling sounds often represent an SBO (choice **C**). Both an ileus and a partial SBO are often treated successfully with bowel rest, administration of intravenous fluids, and nasogastric suction and decompression. Surgical exploration is warranted for cases of obstruction demonstrating progressive distention, evidence of bowel ischemia, fever, leukocytosis, or acidosis.

24

Infections of the Genital Tract

Carolyn Alexander

Please read the following vignette to answer Questions 1–4. A 17-year-old gravida 0, para 0, presents to the emergency department of your hospital with a 2-day history of nausea, vomiting, and lower abdominal pain. She has a history of severe dysmenorrhea since menarche, but her medical and gynecologic history are otherwise unremarkable. On exam she is found to have bilateral lower-quadrant abdominal tenderness, right greater than left, bilateral adnexal tenderness, and a small amount of cervical discharge. Her B-HCG is negative.

1 Each of the following meets the minimum criteria for clinical diagnosis of pelvic inflammatory disease (PID) *except:*

- **A.** Bilateral lower-quadrant tenderness
- **B.** Bilateral adnexal fullness
- **C.** Bilateral adnexal tenderness
- **D.** Cervical motion tenderness

B See discussion following Question 4.

2 All of the following are criteria for hospitalization of patients with acute PID *except:*

A. Pregnancy
B. Nulliparity
C. Severe nausea and vomiting
D. Uncertain diagnosis
E. History of pelvic pain

E See discussion following Question 4.

3 Which of the following are the most common organisms isolated from the fallopian tubes of patients with PID?

A. *Trichomonas vaginalis*
B. Human papilloma virus
C. *Chlamydia trachomatis*
D. Anaerobes

D See discussion following Question 4.

4 Each of the following is true regarding Fitz-Hugh and Curtis syndrome *except*:

A. Acute right upper-quadrant pain
B. Elevated liver enzymes
C. Formation of fibrous perihepatic adhesions
D. Results from the inflammatory process of PID

B In the United States, the majority of PID cases are caused by ascending infection. Endocervical *N. gonorrhoeae* or *C. trachomatis* infections develop and lead to mucosal inflammation. Clinical exam reveals mucopurulent endocervicitis associated with vaginal leukorrhea. The cervical mucus barrier is altered, and access to the endometrial cavity is attained. This process may be facilitated by the gonococci and anaerobes attaching to spermatozoa, which carry them up into the endometrium. When cultures are performed from the fallopian tubes, the most common microorganisms isolated are anaerobes including *Bacteroides* species, *Peptococcus* species, and

Clostridium species. This continuum of infection is associated with signs of inflammation.

The minimum criteria for clinical diagnosis of PID are as follows: bilateral lower abdominal tenderness, cervical motion tenderness, and bilateral adnexal tenderness. Additional criteria for diagnosis include temperature greater than 38°C, abnormal cervical discharge, and elevated erythrocyte sedimentation rate (ESR) or C-reactive protein. An endometrial biopsy may reveal either acute (neutrophilic) or chronic (plasma cell) endomyometritis or evidence of both. Ultrasound may reveal a tuboovarian abscess, which is one of the criteria for hospitalization of patients with acute PID. Other criteria for hospitalization include nulliparity, pregnancy, temperature greater than 38°C, inability to tolerate PO intake, peritoneal signs, failure to respond to oral antibiotics within 48 hours, and uncertain diagnosis.

The Fitz-Hugh and Curtis syndrome is caused by the inflammatory process of PID. It is characterized by fibrous perihepatic adhesions that resemble violin strings. Patients complain of right upper-quadrant pain, but serologic studies reveal no elevation of the liver enzymes. Both *N. gonorrhoeae* and *C. trachomatis* have been isolated from the liver capsule in patients with this syndrome.

Please read the following vignette to answer Questions 5 and 6.

A 32-year-old gravida 3, para 3, seeks your advice about an intrauterine device (IUD) for contraception. She has no medical problems and no history of surgery. She has had 3 uneventful pregnancies and 3 vaginal deliveries, her most recent 4 months ago. She was treated for chlamydia at age 21 and a single abnormal Pap smear at age 28, but otherwise her gynecologic history is unremarkable. Her pelvic exam is normal.

---

5 With regard to IUD insertion and infection, this patient:

A. Is at greatest risk of infection at the time of insertion

B. Is at high risk of infection because of her abnormal Pap smear

C. Is at high risk of infection because of her history of chlamydia

D. Should wait until she is at least 6 months postpartum, to minimize the risk of infection

A See discussion following Question 6.

6 All of the following are true *except:*

A. IUDs are a very effective, long-term, reversible method of birth control.

B. IUDs can be used in patients who are breastfeeding.

C. IUDs are safe in patients who are smokers.

D. IUDs cause frequent infections with actinomycosis.

D Worldwide, approximately 12% of reproductive-age married women use IUDs. In the United States, however, only 0.8% of women using contraception use them. An IUD is a very effective, long-term, reversible method of birth control. They are safe in patients who are smokers or breastfeeding. With regard to IUD insertion and infection, the patient is at greatest risk of infection at the time of insertion. For 21 days after insertion, a transient sixfold increased risk of infection exists, after which the rate of PID decreases to 0.059 per 100 woman-years of use with the Copper T380A device. Sexual behavior and exposure to chlamydia and gonorrhea produce the largest risk for PID. In the current literature, there are no studies evaluating whether the risk of progression to PID is greater in a woman with cervicitis and a modern copper IUD than without one. In spite of this, manufacturer and The American College for Obstetrics and Gynecology recommendations list any lifetime history of PID as a contraindication to use of a copper IUD.

Please read the following vignette to answer Questions 7–9.
A 22-year-old gravida 0, para 0, presents to urgent care complaining of sudden onset of severe, intermittent itching that worsens at night. She states that it is worse in her axillae and groin. She is in excellent health and has never had any

surgery. She is sexually active and has a new partner of 2 weeks. She takes no medications and has no allergies. She admits to smoking half a pack of cigarettes a day, occasional alcohol, and no illicit drugs. On exam, there are multiple vesicles in between her fingers as well as burrows noted on her mons pubis.

---

7 What is the best method of diagnosis?

A. Examine skin scrapings under oil.
B. Perform a culture of the vesicles.
C. Examine KOH preparation.
D. Send serology.

A See discussion following Question 9.

8 What is the best treatment option?

A. Acyclovir
B. Permethrin 5% cream
C. Cortisone
D. Nystatin powder

B See discussion following Question 9.

9 Which of the following is another treatment option?

A. Valcyclovir
B. Ketoconazole
C. 1% γ-benzene hexachloride (lindane)
D. Imiquimod 5% cream

C Human scabies is caused by an insect, *Sarcoptes scabiei.* The female mite excavates a burrow in the skin and lays eggs. It is transmitted sexually or nonsexually via close contact and may infect any part of the body, especially flexural surfaces. Clinically, it manifests itself with an insidious onset of a pruritic, pleomorphic rash. The best method of diagnosis is to examine skin scrapings under oil and identifying the mite, eggs, or fecal pellets. The best treatment is the use of permethrin 5% cream to all areas of the body. Because of reports of resistance to 1% γ-benzene hexachloride or lindane, it should be considered when permethrin is not available. Clothes and linens should be laundered in hot water and heat dried and removed from body contact for 72 hours. In addition, sexual partners should be treated.

Please read the following vignette to answer Questions 10 and 11.

A 20-year-old gravida 1, para 1, presents to your office complaining of frothy, pink vaginal discharge. She has no medical problems and has had one uncomplicated vaginal delivery. On exam, her cervix appears erythematous and friable.

---

10 Which of the following is the most likely finding on wet smear?

A. Multiple hyphae
B. Clue cells
C. Unicellular, flagellated organisms
D. Overgrowth of bacteria

C See discussion following Question 11.

11 Which of the following is the best treatment regimen?

A. Metronidazole, 2 g orally (one dose)
B. Clindamycin phosphate 2% cream (7 days)
C. Trimethoprim/sulfamethoxazole DS, one tab orally (3 days)
D. None of the above

A *Trichomonas vaginalis* is sexually contracted and accounts for approximately 25% of infectious vaginitis. On wet smear it appears as a unicellular, flagellated protozoan that is slightly larger than a white blood cell. The vaginal discharge should have a pH of 5.0–7.0. The ideal treatment is one dose of 2g metronidazole orally. This treatment should be avoided during the first trimester of pregnancy. Alcohol should be avoided as well. Sexual partners must be treated, and patients should be instructed to avoid intercourse until symptoms resolve.

25

Ectopic Pregnancy

Michelle Taylor

1 Which of the following represents the most common tubal implantation sites of an ectopic pregnancy in order of most frequent to least frequent?

- **A.** Isthmus, cornua, fimbriae, ampulla
- **B.** Ampulla, isthmus, cornua, fimbriae
- **C.** Ampulla, isthmus, fimbriae, cornua
- **D.** Fimbriae, cornua, isthmus, ampulla
- **E.** Fimbriae, isthmus, ampulla, cornua

C The vast majority of ectopic pregnancies (EPs) are tubal. Most tubal pregnancies are found in the distal two-thirds of the fallopian tube. The ampulla is the most common site of implantation, accounting for 78% of EPs; 12% are located in the isthmus, 5% in the fimbriae, and 2% are cornual.

2 A 32-year-old gravida 4, para 3013, with a history of a bilateral tubal ligation presents to your office complaining of nausea, vomiting, and abdominal pain for 1 week. Urine pregnancy test is positive. The date of her last menstrual period was 5 weeks ago. You advise the patient to:

- **A.** Register for prenatal care within the next 6–8 weeks.
- **B.** Follow up in 1 week so that you may obtain a serum hCG at that time. If the value is greater than 1,500, she will be scheduled for a pelvic sonogram.

C. Undergo a suction D&C for undesired pregnancy.

D. Go to laboratory for quantitative β-hCG immediately, then report for pelvic sonogram.

D Abdominal pain and amenorrhea are two common symptoms of EP. One-third or more pregnancies occurring after failure of tubal sterilization are likely to be EPs. Appropriate management would include quantitative serum β-hCG and pelvic sonogram immediately, to rule out EP.

3 Which of the following statements regarding treatment for ectopic pregnancy is true?

A. Laparoscopy is the preferred surgical approach to EP in the hemodynamically stable patient.

B. Salpingostomy involves incising the fallopian tubes linearly, removing any products of conception, and then closing the remaining tubal defect.

C. The failure rate after methotrexate therapy is in the range of 70–85%.

D. In women with no infertility factor, studies have shown a slight advantage of salpingectomy over salpingostomy.

A Laparoscopy has become the preferred surgical approach to EP in the hemodynamically stable patient. When performing a salpingostomy, the tubal defect is left open to heal by secondary intention. The success rate after methotrexate therapy is in the range of 70–85%. In women with no history of infertility, studies have shown no difference between salpingectomy and salpingostomy.

4 Contraindications to methotrexate administration include all of the following *except*:

A. Poor patient compliance

B. Fetal cardiac activity

C. Renal disease

D. Active peptic ulcer disease

E. Vaginal bleeding

E All of these are contraindications except for vaginal bleeding. Also included as contraindications are hepatic disease or dysfunction and blood dyscrasias (ex. leukopenia, severe thrombocytopenia).

5 While obtaining preoperative informed consent on your patient with EP, the patient inquires about her subsequent fertility. You advise her:

A. A history of pelvic inflammatory disease is the single most important factor influencing future fertility.

B. In females with a history of infertility, a slightly higher subsequent pregnancy rate and EP rate is found in women who undergo salpingostomy as opposed to salpingectomy.

C. Not to worry—90% of women will conceive after an EP, and there is no effect on overall fertility, regardless of treatment.

D. Recurrent ectopic pregnancies are rare.

B Studies have shown a slightly higher subsequent pregnancy rate and EP rate in women with histories of infertility who undergo salpingostomy as opposed to salpingectomy. A history of previous infertility is the single most important factor influencing future fertility. Only 45–75% of women will conceive after an EP, and of those, approximately 20% will have a recurrent EP.

26

Chronic Pelvic Pain

Francisco Rojas

1 A 31-year-old nulliparous white female goes to the gynecologist complaining of 10 months of progressive abdominal pain, dysmenorrhea, and dyspareunia. She has been married for 2 years, has not used contraception, and has never been pregnant. Past medical history, on the other hand, is unremarkable, and physical exam reveals no abnormalities. The most likely diagnosis is

A. Adenomyosis
B. Endometriosis
C. Leiomyomatosis
D. Interstitial cystitis
E. Irritable bowel syndrome

B Patients with adenomyosis and leiomyomatosis most likely will have abnormal uterine bleeding. Pelvic pain caused by interstitial cystitis will have associated frequency, nocturia, and urgency. In the same way, irritable bowel syndrome presents with history of constipation, bloating, and diarrhea. Among these medical conditions, endometriosis is the most likely to explain menstrual cycle-related pain, progressive intensity, and infertility.

2 In a 31-year-old woman, with regard to causes of chronic pelvic pain, all of the following statements are true *except*:

A. The observation of adhesions is not proof of a cause-and-effect relationship.

B. Endometriosis is found in approximately 10% of women who have had laparoscopy for chronic pelvic pain.

C. Tuberculosis is the most likely cause of chronic pelvic infection.

D. Degeneration of a leiomyoma may cause pain.

E. Ovarian tenderness and postcoital ache are associated with pelvic vein incompetence.

B Chronic pelvic pain can be present without adhesions, and it is common to find adhesions in patients without pain. Tuberculosis and uterine fibroids could explain pelvic pain under specific circumstances. The combination of ovarian point tenderness on abdominal exam and a history of a postcoital ache is 94% sensitive and 77% specific for pelvic vein incompetence. Grossly evident endometriosis is diagnosed in 30–50% of women who undergo laparoscopy for chronic pelvic pain.

3 Concerning the treatment of chronic pelvic pain, all of the following statements are true *except:*

A. Narcotics are contraindicated because of a high risk of addiction.

B. Analgesics will usually only partially alleviate the pain rather than providing complete relief.

C. Low-dose tricyclic antidepressants are associated with constipation and morning drowsiness.

D. Muscular problems are better treated with physical therapy than muscle relaxants.

E. Psychological counseling is important, especially for those patients with a history of sexual or physical abuse.

A Analgesics have a transient palliative effect and should be taken on a regular basis, not as needed, because this regimen provides the greatest degree of pain relief over time. The judicious use of narcotics is reasonable and can greatly improve a patient's ability to function. Antidepressants modify the pain threshold and are especially useful when there are signs of depression. The sedative side effect from muscle relaxants limit their use. Counseling is a necessary part of successful therapy in patients with a history of abuse, and is an often underutilized tool in the treatment of chronic pain.

27

Urogynecology

Renée Ward

1 A 47-year-old gravida 2, para 1011, comes to your office complaining of leaking urine when she coughs or laughs. She voids frequently, every 1–2 hours during the day, but denies nocturia. On exam, you note well-estrogenized tissue, a hypermobile uretha, and a mild cystocele. Which of the following would you do next?

A. Sacral nerve root stimulation

B. Referral to neurology

C. Urodynamic studies

D. Prescribe tolterodine tartrate and bladder-retraining drills

E. Tension-free vaginal tape sling or a Burch procedure

D This patient has symptoms of both stress and urge incontinence. Thirty percent of women with mixed incontinence become dry after nonsurgical therapy alone; thus a trial of tolterodine tartrate or oxybutynin chloride accompanied by bladder-retraining skills is an appropriate first step in treatment. If this is unsuccessful, urodynamic studies can further elucidate the deficits present and guide decisions about invasive treatments, such as a suburethral sling or urethropexy. Unless there is a history of a neurologic disease or a focal neurologic deficit, it is not necessary to obtain additional neurologic studies or a neurology consult. Sacral nerve root stimulation is an invasive procedure for patients with disease that is refractory to other treatments.

2 A 64-year-old woman complains of fecal incontinence after undergoing a posterior vulvectomy for microinvasive vulvar carcinoma. She loses liquid and soft stool on a daily basis, requiring her to use protective undergarments. Anal manometry shows a sphincter deficit from 10 to 2 o'clock. What do you recommend for treatment?

A. Muscle transposition

B. Sphincteroplasty

C. A Marshall-Marchetti-Krantz procedure

D. Pelvic floor exercises

E. Colostomy

B Anal incontinence is a known complication after an extensive vulvectomy. In this case, anal sphincteroplasty will repair the defect. If this is unsuccessful, transposition of the gracilis muscle may be needed to re-create a functional sphincter. If both of these options fail, a colostomy could be used as a last resort. Pelvic floor exercises can help with early fatigability of the sphincter muscle, but are not suitable for the patient with extensive injury to the anal sphincter. Similarly, bulking agents and medications to slow colonic motility can help with less severe forms of incontinence, but are not suitable for an intrinsic sphincter defect. Marshall-Marchetti-Krantz is a retropubic urethropexy procedure for stress urinary incontinence.

3 An 88-year-old woman with poorly controlled diabetes mellitus, congestive heart failure, hypertension, and a history of three-vessel coronary bypass surgery complains of complete procidentia. She has used a pessary in the past, but is unable to tolerate use now due to persistent and recurrent yeast infections. She is not sexually active. What other treatments would you offer her?

A. LeFort partial colpocleisis

B. Total vaginal hysterectomy

C. Total abdominal hysterectomy

D. Hormone replacement therapy with Kegel exercises

A A LeFort partial colpocleisis is an excellent option for a patient who is a poor surgical candidate because it can be performed under regional anesthesia. It is critical to emphasize that the vagina is obliterated and will be nonfunctional. Colpocleisis is an important option to consider in elderly patients who are no longer sexually active with multiple comorbid conditions, because chronic pessary use can lead to ulcerations. Although a total vaginal hysterectomy may not be technically difficult to perform in the setting of complete procidentia, the perioperative risks must be considered. A total abdominal hysterectomy would carry even greater perioperative risks. Complete uterine prolapse cannot be cured with hormonal treatments and pelvic floor exercises.

4 A 28-year-old primigravida at 24 weeks' gestational age requests a primary elective cesarean delivery from her obstetrician. She has read that a vaginal delivery predisposes her to pelvic organ prolapse and incontinence in the future. All of the following are appropriate and correct responses to this patient *except:*

A. Vaginal deliveries can lead to the prolongation of nerve conduction in the pelvic floor, although this resolves in 80% of women.

B. Forceps deliveries are associated with future fecal incontinence. Denervation injury to the sphincter muscle may cause persistent incontinence, even in the setting of a successful anatomic repair of the anal sphincter.

C. Older age is associated with urinary and fecal incontinence for women who have suffered an obstetrical injury.

D. Cesarean delivery has never been shown to be protective of pelvic floor damage. Pregnancy in and of itself may be detrimental to the pelvic floor, regardless of the delivery route.

C Older age is associated with urinary and fecal incontinence, regardless of obstetric injury. The other statements all represent appropriate counseling.

5 A 54-year-old woman presents to your office with Stage II uterovaginal prolapse. On ultrasound a 5-cm simple adnexal cyst is seen. What is your treatment of choice for the pelvic organ prolapse?

A. Sacrospinous ligament suspension
B. Abdominal sacral colpopexy
C. Moschcowitz procedure
D. Halban culdoplasty
E. McCall culdoplasty

B Given the concurrent finding of an adnexal mass, this patient will require an exploratory laparotomy. The preferred method of vaginal suspension from an abdominal approach is an abdominal sacral colpopexy. Sacrospinous ligament suspension provides vaginal apex support, but is performed vaginally. Moschcowitz and Halban culdoplasties are used to repair enteroceles from an abdominal approach, but do not support the vaginal cuff. McCall culdoplasty both corrects an enterocele and provides apical support for the vagina, but is performed vaginally.

28

Fertility Control

Julia Cron

1 A healthy 33-year-old gravida 4, para 3103, has just delivered via an uncomplicated spontaneous delivery after an unremarkable prenatal course. She is planning on breastfeeding. She may consider having more children in the future. She would like to discuss contraceptive options with you. Which of the following would not be appropriate for her?

A. Progestin-only birth control pills

B. Combination birth control pills

C. Intrauterine device (IUD)

D. Condoms

E. Laparoscopic tubal ligation

E Nonhormonal contraceptives are the contraceptive of choice for breastfeeding women. These would include condoms, an IUD (which may be inserted at the 6-week postpartum visit), and tubal ligation (which would not be an option in this woman, who desires future fertility). Progestin-only contraceptives (injectibles, pills, and implants) have only a theoretical impact on milk letdown, and there are no documented adverse effects on infants. Therefore, these are the preferred forms of postpartum hormonal contraception. Combination oral contraceptive pills may be used by breastfeeding women after breastfeeding has been well established (ACOG recommends 6 weeks postpartum).

2 Match the clinical situation with the best contraceptive option:

1. Combined oral contraceptive (COC) pills
2. Tubal ligation
3. Condoms
4. Depo-Provera
5. Levonorgestrel IUD

A. 37-year-old para 2012 with no medical problems and undesired future fertility

B. 17-year-old para 2032 with a recent admission for pelvic inflammatory disease

C. 28-year-old para 1001 with a history of menorrhagia and dysmenorrhea and a history of deep venous thrombosis with her pregnancy

D. 21-year-old para 2012 who became pregnant while on COCs because she was unable to remember to take her pills every day

E. 20-year-old with metorrhagia and no other medical problems

1, E COCs are effective contraceptives and can often regulate irregular menses.
2, A Surgical sterilization, including tubal ligation, is an extremely effective contraceptive method and the only permanent method available.
3, B Condoms are the only effective contraceptive device to protect against sexually transmitted diseases including gonorrhea and chlamydia, common causes of pelvic inflammatory disease (PID). In this patient, a backup contraceptive method such as Depo-Provera or COCs may be recommended.
4, D Depo-Provera has the advantage over COCs that it does not require patient action every day. For this reason, its perfect use and average use effectiveness are the same. In contrast, the average use effectiveness of COCs is significantly less than its perfect use effectiveness.
5, C COCs would be contraindicated in this patient, given her history of deep vein thrombosis. The levonorgestrel IUD is advantageous over other IUDs because it is associated with fewer side effects and may decrease previously existing menstrual irregularities.

3 Match the three major U.S. Supreme Court rulings on elective termination of pregnancy:

1. *Roe v. Wade,* 1973
2. *Planned Parenthood v. Casey,* 1992
3. *Stenberg v. Carhart,* 2000

A. Women, in consultation with their physicians, have a constitutional right to abortion up until the time of fetal viability.

B. A Nebraska law that restricted late-term abortions was unconstitutional, as it was too broad and did not contain an exception to protect the health of the mother.

C. A woman's right to abortion was upheld, but states have the right to enact restrictions that do not create an "undue burden" for women.

1, A; 2, C; 3, B

4 A 34-year-old para 1011 presents for her postpartum visit. She is breastfeeding without difficulty, but supplementing with formula because the baby always seems hungry. She has not been sexually active and has not had a menstrual period since her delivery. With reference to the lactational amenorrhea method (LAM) of contraception, the use of formula may increase her risk of getting pregnant.

A. True

B. False

A **True.** In order for LAM to be effective, certain criteria must be met. Feeding must be at least every 4 hours during the day and every 6 hours at night. Supplemental feeding should not exceed 5–10% of the total feedings. The pregnancy rate is still 2% in the first 6 months postpartum and 6% from 6 months to 1 year postpartum.

5 A 16-year-old nullipara presents with questions regarding emergency contraception (EC). She reports that she had unprotected intercourse less than 24 hours ago and does not desire a pregnancy. Considering the situation and potential side effects, which is the best option for this patient?

A. Wait for her menstrual period to come

B. Combination (estrogen and progesterone) emergency contraceptive pills such as Preven

C. Progesterone-only emergency contraceptive pills such as Plan B

D. Placement of an IUD

C Currently, there are several options for emergency hormonal contraception. Preven is a prepackaged product that contains four pills of 0.25 mg levonorgestrel and 0.05 mg ethinyl estradiol, taken in two doses 12 hours apart. Plan B contains one 0.75-mg levonorgestrel pill repeated in 12 hours, and has been shown to have an improved side-effect profile over Preven (less nausea, breast tenderness, etc.) while being equally effective. Both medications should be taken within 72 hours of unprotected intercourse for an effectiveness rate of approximately 98%. An IUD may also be inserted within 5 days of unprotected intercourse for an effectiveness rate of approximately 99%, but this is most likely overly invasive for this 16-year-old girl.

29

Sexual Assault and Domestic Violence

Wendy Monthy

1 A 17-year-old gravida 1, para 0, at 33-1/7 weeks' gestation is brought by her boyfriend to Labor and Delivery after a fall. She complains of abdominal pain and decreased fetal movement since the accident. While taking the patient's history, it is important to do all of the following *except:*

A. Determine the cause of the fall, making certain to ask about domestic violence as a possibility.

B. Ask her boyfriend to leave the room, to ensure privacy during the interview.

C. Ask about a history of previous trauma, chronic pain, or psychological distress.

D. Use terms such as "abused" and "battered" when asking about domestic violence, as these are the most direct terms.

D Screening for domestic violence is an important role for a physician. This involves asking about domestic violence as a part of a routine patient evaluation during office visits and emergency room evaluations. Studies show that women who were asked about violence more than once during pregnancy report higher prevalence rates, so it is important to ask periodically during prenatal care. In addition, the patient should be interviewed in private. The interviewer should avoid being judgmental or using value-laden terms such as "abused" or "battered." Be certain to ask specific questions regarding prior emergency room visits for injury. In addition, these patients may report difficulty with chronic pain or psychological disorders more frequently.

2 Which of the following statements regarding sexual assault and domestic violence is *false*?

A. Women are more likely to be injured, raped, or even killed by a current or former male partner than by all other types of assailants combined.

B. Up to 12% of U.S. women in an ongoing relationship experience some type of violence each year.

C. Violence occurs in up to 20–37% of pregnancies and is more prevalent than common obstetric disorders such as preeclampsia, gestational diabetes, and placenta previa.

D. The risk of acquiring HIV infection from a sexual assault is about 10%.

D Although some women are victims of an acute attack or rape, the majority find themselves in long-standing abusive relationships, which tend to develop into a cycle of violent episodes followed by a period of apologies. This cycle progressively escalates into more violent episodes. Escape from the relationship is difficult. Battering may begin or escalate during pregnancy and can result in poor pregnancy outcomes, including miscarriage, preterm labor, or low birthweight. When the episode of violence includes an element of sexual assault, it is important to treat presumptively for sexually transmitted diseases (STDs), because approximately 43% of sexual assault victims have at least one preexisting STD. The risk of acquiring an STD from an assault is as follows: gonorrhea 6–12%, syphilis 3%, and HIV infection <1%.

3 After the boyfriend of the patient in Question 1 leaves the room, she confides in her doctor that in fact she was punched in her abdomen and pushed to the ground by her boyfriend. She also reports that this is a recurrent problem and she is ready to make a change for the safety of her fetus. She asks for help in making an exit plan. A successful exit plan should include:

A. Packing a change of clothes and an extra set of house and car keys to be kept next to the door for a quick departure.

B. Gradually taking small amounts of cash from her partner's wallet without him noticing, so she will have enough money once she is gone.

C. Deciding upon a plan of exactly where to go, regardless of the time, day or night.

D. Creating false identification papers such as birth certificate, driver's license, and Social Security card so that she may not be tracked by her boyfriend.

C In empowering a victim of domestic violence, it is important to review with her an exit plan or exit drill. The following exit plan has been proposed for a woman who feels that she or her children are in danger from her male partner: Have a change of clothes packed, and an extra set of house or car keys. These can be placed in a suitcase and stored with a friend or neighbor. Cash, a checkbook, and a savings account book may also be kept with the individual chosen. Identification papers should be kept available for school enrollment, financial assistance, etc. Something of special interest to each child should be taken. A plan of exactly where to go should be decided upon, including a friend or relative's home or a shelter.

30

Pediatric Gynecology

Andrea C. Nugent
Lisa Kolp

1 It is Memorial Day weekend and your hospital has a scaled-down staff. A 16-year-old girl presents to you who has never menstruated and who has abdominal pain and low-grade fever. She also has had a sore throat for the last 2 days. She experienced thelarche at 12 years of age, andrenarche at age 13 years. On physical examination, she has Tanner stage IV breasts and pubic hair. Pelvic exam reveals normal external genitalia but no palpable vagina. The next best diagnostic tool would be

A. Pelvic CT scan

B. Pelvic ultrasound

C. Pelvic MRI

D. Examination under anesthesia

B This patient has primary amenorrhea, likely due to vaginal agenesis versus outflow obstruction. Her Tanner stage IV breast and pubic hair demonstrate likely normal ovarian estrogen secretion. The next step is to determine whether she has a uterus or vagina present. If no vagina is present, this is consistent with Mayer-Rokitansky-Küster-Hauser syndrome or congenital absence of the uterus and vagina. If the uterus is present, obstruction may be evident and, with the coexisting fevers, she may become septic. Therefore, the best method of ascertaining this is via a pelvic ultrasound. This procedure is minimally invasive and may enable you to see a distended endometrial cavity resulting from hematometrocolpos, which may be seen either with imperforate hymen or transverse vaginal septum. Pelvic CT could show you the presence or absence of the uterus/vagina; however, it may not lend to easy visualization of the endometrium and may not be available because of the limited availability of staff. A pelvic MRI is useful to delineate tissue planes and to evaluate uterine anomalies such as uterine didelphys. Because of its expense and limited availability, an MRI would not be the next best diagnostic tool. Finally, an examination under anesthesia would not definitively ascertain whether a uterus was present. However, if, on Valsalva maneuver, a bulging membrane is seen, an imperforate hymen is likely to be the diagnosis.

2 You are the resident on call and are asked to consult on a 2-week-old infant. She was brought to the pediatric emergency department because of diarrhea. On investigation, an abdominal ultrasound was performed and a 3-cm adnexal mass was found. The mass appears cystic in nature, without any solid components. The child is in a flexed position and sleeping quietly. You recommend

A. Consult by pediatric surgery for immediate laparotomy

B. Admission for observation and serial sonography

C. Transabdominal aspiration of the cyst

B The fetus at term may develop ovarian cysts due to stimulation of their ovarian tissue by maternal estrogen. Most of these cysts will resolve spontaneously within 4–6 weeks of birth. Malignancy is exceedingly rare in this group, and these cysts should usually be followed with serial sonography. Torsion can be of concern, especially with cysts larger than 4 cm. Symptoms of torsion in this age group may include pain, gastrointestinal (GI) disturbance, or irritability. Because of this baby's GI disturbance, admission for observation is recommended, as it may also be a symptom of torsion. If the child appeared to be in pain (e.g., inconsolable crying, with knees drawn up to the chest), a pediatric surgery consult might be in order. However, the child is resting comfortably. Transabdominal cyst aspiration is not recommended for a 3-cm cyst, as the risk of injury to surrounding structures (bowel, bladder, vessels, etc.) would outweigh the benefit of draining a cyst that is likely to resolve if managed conservatively.

3 A 9-year-old girl was taken to the emergency department by her father after falling off her bunk bed onto a wooden rocking horse below. She has since been unable to urinate because of burning for the last 12 hours. On physical examination, she has a large ecchymosis at the anterior portion of the labia minora and clitoris. The urethra is swollen and bruised. There is no obvious disturbance of the posterior fourchette or vagina. She will not allow a speculum to be passed or a urinary catheter. Her hematocrit is within normal limits. The best management for the patient is

A. Examination under anesthesia with passage of a urinary catheter

B. Warm compresses and observation

C. Call the Child Protective Services to report likely sexual abuse

D. Despite the child's crying and resistance, insert a urinary catheter

A Because of the anterior location of the injury, it is likely that she has a straddle injury due to her fall. The inability to pass urine for 12 hours necessitates a urinary catheter. She is resistant to catheterization, so to force a urinary catheter may traumatize the patient and lend to fear of future pelvic exams. Therefore, an examination under anesthesia is warranted to pass the urinary catheter. In addition, an examination under anesthesia will also allow a more thorough examination to ascertain if any penetrative injuries were incurred. If the child was able to urinate and less time had passed without urination, warm compresses and observation would be appropriate management. Finally, calling Child Protective Services would be inappropriate with the amount of information given. If the injury was posterior in location, one might be more suspicious. If any definitive findings of sexual abuse were present (see Table 30-2 in the *Johns Hopkins Manual of Gynecology and Obstetrics*, 2nd edition, page 359), one might consider this option.

4 A 6-year-old girl presents to clinic with her mother complaining of vulvar pain and itching as well as a foul-smelling discharge from the vagina for 3 weeks. She is given a bubble bath every night before bed. On physical examination, both labia majora and minora are erythematous. Stool can be seen in the labial folds. There is no obvious disturbance of the hymenal tissues or vagina. You educate the patient and her parent on hygiene issues and instruct her to stop bubble baths. The most likely pathogen is

A. *Chlamydia*

B. *Monilia*

C. *Gardnerella vaginalis*

D. *Staphylococcus aureus*

D As there is no evidence of sexual abuse, *Chlamydia* and *Gardnerella vaginalis* are unlikely pathogens in this child. *Monilia* is likely to demonstrate satellite lesions, which will make diagnosis easier. In addition, not common in this age group is a vulvar pathogen. For this reason, the most likely pathogen would be superinfection of the irritated vulvar tissues with *Staphylococcus aureus*.

5 An 8-year-old girl presents to your clinic. Her mother tells you that she looks “abnormal down below.” On further questioning, you find out that over the last month she has grown pubic hair. On physical examination, you notice that the girl’s voice is much deeper than one would expect for an 8-year-old. She has scattered pubic hair and evidence of virilization of the clitoris. As a part of the workup, a pelvic ultrasound is obtained. An adnexal mass is noted that is suspicious for malignancy. Which type of ovarian tumor is it most likely to be?

A. Granulosa cell tumor

B. Immature teratoma

C. Epithelial adenocarcinoma

D. Arrhenoblastoma

D Arrhenoblastoma is the most common virilizing ovarian tumor in the pediatric patient, although it is a rare tumor overall. A granulosa cell tumor is likely to have estrogenic, rather than androgenic effects. Teratomas are the most common neoplasm in this age group, but an immature teratoma is less common and would not be likely to create androgenic effects. Finally, epithelial adenocarcinoma is very rare in this age group and would be more common in the adult age ranges.

31

Infertility and Assisted Reproductive Technologies

Brandon Bankowski
Nikos Vlahos

Please read the following vignette to answer Questions 1 and 2.

A 40-year-old married woman, gravida 1, para 0, presents to you with a 10-month history of infertility. She has experienced irregular menses for the last 3 years and has experienced withdrawal bleeding in response to several progesterone challenges. Her last menstrual period was 6 weeks ago. She was pregnant at age 17, but the pregnancy was terminated without complication. Her hysterosalpingogram (HSG) was normal several months ago. For the last 3 months she has taken clomiphene citrate during menstrual cycle days 5–9 but has not conceived. Her physician counseled her that she should ask about *in vitro* fertilization.

---

1 With regard to this patient's diagnosis:

A. She should come back in 2 months, when she meets the definition of infertility.

B. She is too young to be in menopause.

C. Even with a normal HSG, she may have "cervical factor" infertility.

D. She may have Asherman's syndrome from the pregnancy termination.

E. "Age factor" does not affect fertility until a woman is in her mid-40s.

C The strict definition of infertility is failure to conceive after 1 year of regular intercourse without contraception. While this patient does not quite meet the time requirement, since the fertility of a 39-year-old woman is decreased simply because of her age, evaluation and potential treatment should proceed without delay. Age-related infertility, which is due to oocyte abnormalities and decreased ovarian reserve, is increasing in many cultures because of the social trends to delay childbearing. Data from the American Society for Reproductive Medicine (ASRM) (Figure 31.1) demonstrate that infertility, even after *in vitro* fertilization (IVF), becomes more pronounced after the age of 35.

Menopause is defined clinically as the cessation of menstrual periods for 1 year. The average age of

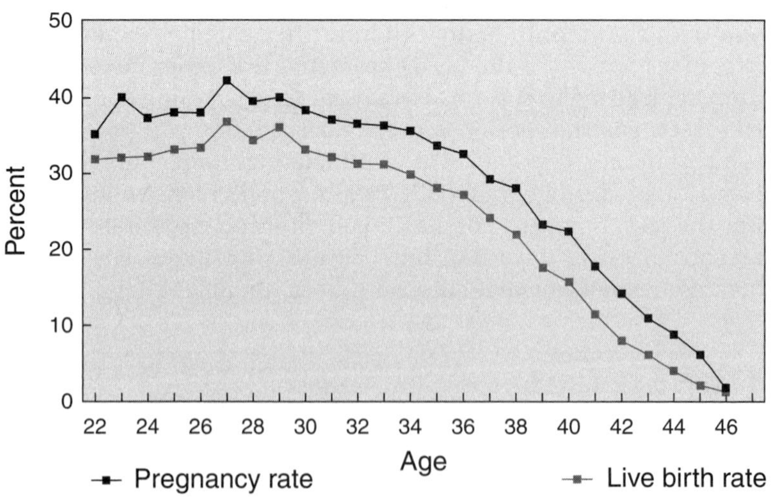

FIGURE 31.1 (*Source:* Centers for Disease Control and Prevention, American Society for Reproductive Medicine, Society for Assisted Reproductive Technology, RESOLVE 1999 Assisted Reproductive Technology Success Rates, Atlanta, GA: Centers for Disease Control and Prevention, 2001.)

menopause in the United States is approximately 51 years with a range of ±7 years. Although this patient is outside this range, she may be experiencing "perimenopause," which may last for 4 or 5 years as the patient transitions into the ovarian failure associated with menopause. Premature ovarian failure is defined as menopause before the age of 35.

An HSG is designed to evaluate the cervix, endometrial cavity, and fallopian tubes. Although cervical stenosis may be visualized, abnormalities of the cervical mucus associated with clomiphene citrate use cannot be diagnosed on an HSG.

Asherman's syndrome is characterized by severe endometrial adhesions that often obliterate the outflow tract for menstrual blood, leading to secondary amenorrhea. Although this syndrome may occur after a D&C for a pregnancy termination, the patient's menstrual history and HSG are not suggestive of this condition.

2 At this time, further recommendations may include each of the following tests *except:*

A. A semen analysis

B. Laparoscopy

C. Thyroid Stimulating Hormone (TSH) and prolactin

D. Baseline (menstrual cycle day 2 or 3) follicle stimulating hormone (FSH)

B The differential diagnosis of infertility includes male factors (30%); ovarian factors and anovulation (25%); structural factors that affect the fallopian tubes, uterus, or peritoneum (such as endometriosis) (25%); cervical factors (10%); and unexplained factors. Because a couple may have more than one reason for being infertile, a semen analysis is a critical part of the infertility workup. A male partner with azospermia or severe oligospermia may require testicular biopsy, intracytoplasmic sperm injection (ICSI), or even sperm donation instead of standard IVF in order to achieve a successfully fertilized embryo.

A laparoscopy is the most invasive portion of the infertility evaluation. Although this patient does not have the luxury of time because of her age, she should still have a thorough basic evaluation consisting of the less invasive and less expensive tests before undergoing surgery.

The laboratory tests mentioned (basal FSH, TSH, prolactin) are useful, inexpensive, and minimally invasive methods to evaluate ovarian reserve and possible treatable causes of the oligomenorrhea that may be contributing to the infertility.

3 Before proceeding to assisted reproductive technologies, an infertile patient should undergo treatment for medical problems that may have a negative impact on a patient's fertility. All of the following conditions/behaviors may affect the fertility of a couple *except:*

A. Hyperprolactinemia
B. Hypothyroidism
C. Marathon training
D. Hyperthyroidism
E. Weight-bearing exercise
F. Smoking

E A variety of conditions can disrupt reproduction in a human couple. In addition to structural abnormalities of the uterus or fallopian tubes, these conditions include problems of the thyroid, pituitary, or ovary. Even behaviors such as excessive exercise or extreme weight gain or loss can interfere with the normal secretion of GnRH from the hypothalamus and thus lead to ovulatory dysfunction. It has been demonstrated that resection or ablation of even minimal endometriosis may enhance fecundity in infertile women. There are no data showing a negative effect of moderate weight-bearing exercise on fertility.

4 If the patient proceeds to *in vitro* fertilization, she may be exposed to a number of different drugs as part of her treatment. Which of the following pairs of drugs and their associated description is *incorrect*?

A. Human chorionic gonadotropin (hCG)—used to simulate the luteinizing hormone (LH) surge

B. GnRH antagonist—causes a flare-up effect that blocks LH secretion and premature luteinization

C. Progesterone—used as supplementation in cases of luteal phase deficiency

D. Clomiphene citrate—oral nonsteroidal compound that may compete with estrogen for estrogen receptor-binding sites

B HCG, which has similar physical properties to LH, is used to simulate the LH surge and leads to final oocyte maturation prior to the oocyte retrieval. Retrieval of the oocytes is scheduled for approximately 34–36 hours after hCG administration in order to avoid retrieving immature oocytes as well as a spontaneous ovulation.

GnRH antagonists are advantageous in that they suppress premature luteinization without causing a flare-up effect.

Progesterone may be used in oral, vaginal, or intramuscular form for supplementation of the luteal phase and corpus luteum until the placenta takes over the production of progesterone at approximately 12 weeks of gestation.

Clomiphene citrate is a synthetic nonsteroidal geometric isomer with mainly antiestrogenic effects and some estrogenic effects. Clomiphene is believed to stimulate ovulation through an antiestrogenic influence on the hypothalamus.

32

Repeated Pregnancy Loss

Ruchi Garg

1 A 26-year-old woman gravida 1, para 0010 has recently had a miscarriage. She is trying to get some answers from her obstetrician with regard to why this occurred. Her physician should explain that the most common type of chromosomal abnormality associated with spontaneous abortions is

A. Turner's (45X)

B. Trisomy

C. Translocation

D. Inversion

E. Mosaicism

B Chromosomal abnormalities are a common cause of spontaneous abortions. In up to 70% of first-trimester miscarriages, a chromosomal abnormality is shown when fetal tissue is tested. These abnormalities include aneuploidies, trisomies, monosomies, etc. Trisomies are the most common type and are detected in almost 50% of miscarriages. The most common trisomies are 13, 16, 18, 21, and 22. The next most common abnormality is 45X (Turner's), which accounts for 25% of all chromosomal abnormalities. Parental chromosomal abnormalities are seen in 3–8% of cases of repeated pregnancy loss (RPL).

Balanced translocation is the most common abnormality found in karyotypes of parents with RPL. Often, the parent is phenotypically normal. Other parental chromosomal abnormalities include inversions and mosaicism.

2 A 29-year-old woman gravida 5, para 0, has been attempting to get pregnant but is experiencing RPL. She has a history of multiple dilation and curettages secondary to elective abortions during her younger years. Her reproductive endocrinologist believes that she might have Asherman's syndrome. Acquired anatomic abnormalities include all of the following *except:*

A. Leiomyomata

B. Intrauterine synechiae

C. *In utero* diethylstilbestrol (DES) exposure

D. Septate uterus

E. Cervical incompetence

D Septate uterus is the most common "congenital" uterine abnormality. Anatomic reasons for RPL can be divided into congenital and acquired problems. Congenital problems include a variety of conditions that often involve Müllerian developmental defects. These losses most commonly occur during the second trimester, although losses at earlier gestational age can also occur. Common uterine abnormalities include septate, bicornuate, didelphic, and less commonly, unicornuate uteri. A septate uterus results from failure of resorption of the paramesonephric ducts and is often associated with poor obstetric outcome. With surgical correction, pregnancy rates have been improved from 15–28% to 80%. Acquired anatomic abnormalities such as submucosal fibroids (unfavorable for implantation), intrauterine synechiae (secondary to instrumentation of the uterus or estrogen deficiency), DES exposure (causes multiple anatomic abnormalities), and cervical incompetence (painless cervical dilation that may be congenital or acquired from a history of cervical surgery such as conization) can all lead to RPL.

3 Match the following letters with the corresponding number:

A. Repeated pregnancy loss	**1.** Detected in 50% of all spontaneous abortions (SABs)
B. Trisomies	**2.** 15% of women with RPL have this
C. Turner's (45X)	**3.** Affects 0.5–1.0% of pregnant women
D. Anatomic abnormality such as septate uteri	**4.** 27% of women with history of losses
E. Autoimmune factors	**5.** Accounts for 25% of all chromosomal abnormalities

A—3 RPL is defined as three consecutive spontaneous abortions before 20 weeks gestation. RPL can be divided into primary, in women without a previous liveborn, and secondary, in those women with at least one prior liveborn infant. Of all clinically documented pregnancies, 15–20% result in spontaneous abortion.

B—1 Trisomies are the most common type of chromosomal abnormality associated with RPL cases.

C—5 Turner's (45X) is the second most common type of chromosomal abnormality associated with RPL, after trisomies.

D—4 Congenital anatomic abnormalities such as septate uteri account for a significant portion of RPL cases.

E—2 Immunologic disorders associated with RPL can be divided into autoimmune and alloimmune factors. Fifteen percent of women with RPL have recognizable autoimmune factors. The most common antibodies include anticardiolipin and lupus anticoagulant.

4 Fill in the blanks with the words provided:

Anticardiolipin	First
Lupus anticoagulant	Second
Anti-SS	Third
Anti-Ro	Anti-la
Factor V Leiden	

The most common antibodies include ______ and ______, which cause thrombosis *in vitro*. *In vivo*, they may cause thrombosis and placental infarctions, which in turn may result in spontaneous abortion in the _______ trimester.

A The most common antibodies (autoimmune factors) include anticardiolipin and lupus anticoagulant, which cause thrombosis *in vitro. In vivo*, they may cause thrombosis and placental infarctions, which in turn may result in spontaneous abortion in the second trimester.

5 A couple has been diagnosed with infertility. A markedly high prevalence of *Mycoplasma hominis* was detected in the cervical mucus and semen of this infertile couple. The appropriate management at this time would be

A. Doxycycline 100 mg BID × 10 days
B. Azithromycin 1 g orally × 1
C. Penicillin 5 million units × 1
D. Gentamycin 80 mg TID × 10 days

A When an infection is diagnosed, the appropriate antibiotic therapy should be instituted. Infections with *Mycoplasma hominis* (a pleuropneumonia-like organism) and *Ureaplasma urealyticum* have been implicated in recurrent abortion and salpingitis. They are treated with 100 mg doxycycline twice daily by mouth for 10 days. Clindamycin, 300 mg three times daily by mouth for 7–10 days, can be used for patients who are pregnant or who are allergic to doxycycline. Appropriate management of this case would be to treat both partners.

33

Uterine Leiomyomas

Kim Bernard

Please read the following vignette to answer Questions 1 and 2.

A 36-year-old gravida 4, para 3003, presents to your office for her annual examination. Since her last visit her menstrual cycle bleeding has been getting heavier and lasting longer. Her menstrual cycles are still regular, but they last 10–14 days. She is very tired and weak. She has had to take days off from work because of the heavy bleeding, but she has not felt the need to be seen by a physician. She denies any pain, pressure, or urinary symptoms. She has no medical problems. Her only surgery was a tubal ligation 5 years ago, and a pregnancy test is negative.

On examination her vital signs are within normal limits. Abdominal exam reveals a palpable mass in the lower abdomen about 3 cm below the umbilicus. On pelvic examination she has normal external genitalia. The cervix has a parous os and is free of lesions and discharge. Vaginal epithelium is without lesions. Bimanual examination reveals an 18-week-size irregular uterus with good mobility and no tenderness. No adnexal masses are appreciated.

---

1 What would be the most appropriate next step in management diagnosis?

A. Pelvic sonogram

B. Total abdominal hysterectomy (TAH)

C. Computed tomography (CT) scan

D. Intravenous pyelogram (IVP)

E. Repeat pelvic in 3 months

A A pelvic sonogram is the most common tool for confirming the diagnosis of leiomyomas. Magnetic resonance imagining (MRI) can be useful in differentiating leiomyomas from other uterine pathology and determining location of fibroids. IVP is not needed unless the patient has obstructive symptoms or hydroureter is seen on ultrasound. Observation without any intervention will likely lead to further symptoms and worsening anemia. An immediate TAH is too aggressive, and should not be the next step in management. The patient needs a complete evaluation and confirmed diagnosis before deciding on an appropriate treatment. A CT scan is not the first imaging modality used for a pelvic mass.

2 A patient's blood work results reveals a hematocrit of 24%. Pelvic ultrasound indicates the presence of a 14-cm pedunculated fundal fibroid with numerous smaller submucosal fibroids. What is the best treatment for this patient?

A. Total abdominal hysterectomy with bilateral salpingo-oophroectomy

B. Blood transfusion

C. Uterine artery embolization (UAE)

D. GnRH agonist for 3 months

E. Myomectomy

D This patient would benefit from a 3-month course of GnRH agonist therapy before surgical treatment. The benefits of this approach are a decrease in uterine size and induction of amenorrhea, allowing the patient to restore her hemoglobin to a normal level and making surgical treatment easier. A TAH and myomectomy are both reasonable surgical options after a trial of suppressive therapy. The patient is not interested in future fertility and has no contraindications to surgery; therefore an abdominal hysterectomy is the surgical option of choice. Bilateral salpingo-oopherectomy should be performed only if significant ovarian pathology is found. Multiple myomectomies have increased risk of larger blood loss, longer operating time, greater postoperative morbidity, and longer hospital stays than hysterectomies. Of patients undergoing myomectomy, 20–25% eventually require a subsequent operation for recurrence. Blood transfusion is not needed, because the patient is asymptomatic. UAE may also be an option. Premature ovarian failure has resulted from UAE, so for this patient a TAH remains the preferable option. Furthermore, UAE is not indicated in a patient with a pedunculated fibroid or one that is >8 cm.

34

Endometriosis

Amy Hearne

Please read the following vignette to answer Questions 1–3. A 24-year-old gravida 2, para 1011, presents to the office with pelvic pain and dysmenorrhea. Pelvic exam reveals nodularity of the uterosacral ligaments. A laparoscopy reveals lesions that are consistent with endometriosis.

---

1 All of the following are found on clinical examination of patients with endometriosis *except:*

A. Nodularity of the inguinal ligaments

B. Tender adnexa

C. Tender swelling of the rectovaginal septum

D. Normal exam

A In many women with endometriosis, no abnormalities are found on examination. Some physical findings associated with endometriosis include nodularity and tenderness of the uterosacral ligaments, tender adnexa, painful swelling of the rectovaginal septum, and fixed retroverted uterus.

2 Which of the following is diagnostic of endometriosis?

A. Blue-black powder-burn lesions visualized at the time of laparoscopy

B. Allen-Masters syndrome

C. Pelvic ultrasound with adnexal mass suspicious for endometrioma

D. Histologic tissue that reveals endometrial glands and stroma

E. Elevated CA-125

D A definitive diagnosis of endometriosis can only be made through histologic exam that reveals ectopic endometrial glands and stroma. Laparoscopy often reveals suspicious lesions that can be biopsied for histologic diagnosis. Lesions may be "classic" blue-black powder-burn lesions or "nonclassic" red, white, tan, nonpigmented, or vesicular lesions. Allen-Masters syndrome is a defect in the peritoneum often scarring overlying endometrial implants. Pelvic ultrasonography can reveal adnexal masses that are suggestive of endometrioma. CA-125 has been elevated in patients with endometriosis, but is not specific for endometriosis.

3 A patient returns for her postoperative checkup. The pathology from the cul-de-sac biopsy of the suspicious lesion revealed endometrial glands and stroma. The patient would like to know what caused her problem. Which of the following is not considered a possible etiology of endometriosis?

A. Retrograde menstuation (Sampson's theory)

B. Environmental factors

C. Coelomic metaplasia

D. Immunologic factors

B The exact etiology of endometriosis is unknown, and all listed are theories of the etiology of endometriosis. Sampson's theory describes retrograde menstruation of endometrial tissue via the fallopian tubes into the peritoneal cavity. Genetic factors are thought to be involved, with an estimated sevenfold higher incidence of endometriosis in women who have a first-degree relative with endometriosis. Environmental factors have not been shown to cause endometriosis. The coelomic metaplasia theory proposes that coelomic epithelium transforms into endometriotic tissue. Immunologic factors involve alterations in the peritoneal cell population. Another theory involves biochemical factors.

35

Amenorrhea

Julie Huh

1 Which of these statements regarding early growth and development is true?

A. Primary amenorrhea refers to the absence of menarche by age 14.

B. Secondary amenorrhea refers to the absence of menses for 3 months after having established regular menses.

C. Adrenarche refers to axillary and pubic hair development and usually occurs after thelarche.

D. An evaluation of amenorrhea may be undertaken if there is no breast development by age 11.

C Adrenarche refers to axillary and pubic hair development and occurs, on average, at 11 years of age. Thelarche refers to breast development and occurs, on average, at 10.8 years of age. Primary amenorrhea refers to the absence of menses by age 16, whereas secondary amenorrhea refers to the absence of menses for 6 months after establishing regular menses. An evaluation of amenorrhea may be undertaken if there is no breast development by age 14, if sexual ambiguity or virilization is present, or if the patient or patient's family is concerned.

2 Which of the following tests is not typically included in the initial workup of secondary amenorrhea?

A. Thyroid-stimulating hormone (TSH) level

B. Prolactin level

C. Progestin challenge

D. Pelvic sonogram

D Pelvic sonogram is not typically included in the initial workup of secondary amenorrhea. Hyperprolactinemia may result in amenorrhea, usually with galactorrhea. Hypothyroidism is associated with amenorrhea. Bleeding in an amenorrheic patient after progestin challenge confirms the presence of estrogen.

3 If withdrawal bleed fails to occur within 10 days of a progestin challenge test, which of the following statements is correct?

A. Exogenous estrogen should be administered, followed by the addition of a progestin agent.

B. This defines the diagnosis of anovulation.

C. It is possible to rule out hypoestrogenemia.

D. Another progestin challenge should be performed.

A Exogenous estrogen can be administered, in the form of 1.25 mg conjugated estrogens or 2 mg estradiol, daily for 21 days. This is followed by 10 mg medroxyprogesterone acetate orally during the last 5 days, to induce withdrawal bleeding. If bleeding occurs, the cause of inadequate estrogen production needs to be elucidated. A positive progestin challenge test may indicate anovulation. Failure to induce uterine bleeding may imply hypoestrogenemia. Another progestin challenge test is not warranted.

4 Which of the following statements regarding gonadal dysgenesis is correct?

A. Approximately one-quarter of patients with gonadal dysgenesis exhibit a mosaic karyotype or a structural abnormality of the X chromosome.

B. In individuals with a Y chromosome, gonadectomy is not recommended because of a low incidence of dysgerminoma and gonadoblastoma.

C. Turner's syndrome (45, XO) is the single most common karyotype found in cases of spontaneous abortion.

D. Patients with pure gonadal dysgenesis may present with primary amenorrhea, eunuchoid habitus, short stature, and infantile internal and external female genitalia.

C Turner's syndrome is the single most common karyotype found in cases of spontaneous abortion, and fewer than 0.3% of affected fetuses survive to term. Approximately one-half of patients with gonadal dysgenesis exhibit a mosaic karyotype or a structural abnormality of the X chromosome. Individuals with a Y chromosome should undergo gonadectomy because a 20% incidence of dysgerminoma and gonadoblastoma exists. Patients with pure gonadal dysgenesis generally have normal stature.

5 All of the following statements regarding hyperprolactinemia are correct *except:*

A. Women with persistent hyperprolactinemia, especially associated with amenorrhea or galactorrhea, or both, should undergo radiographic evaluation.

B. Treatment with a dopamine agonist may help normalize prolactin levels and restore cyclical ovulation.

C. Prolactin secretion is inhibited by dopamine and thyrotropin-releasing hormone (TRH).

D. With elevated prolactin level, thyroid function should be evaluated.

C Hyperprolactinemia may be caused by pituitary micro- or macroadenomas, which may be visualized by CT scan of the head. Abnormally high prolactin levels may be treated with a dopamine agonist, which, in addition to normalizing serum levels, restores menstrual cyclicity. Prolactin secretion is inhibited by dopamine, but secretion of the hormone is stimulated by serotonin and thyrotropin-releasing hormone. Primary hypothyroidism may produce elevated TRH and thus elevated prolactin.

36

Abnormal Uterine Bleeding

Betty Chou

1 A 45-year-old obese woman who has a known history of fibroids is referred to you by her primary care physician for evaluation of her symptoms of vaginal bleeding. She states that her menstrual cycles are becoming more irregular, with very heavy bleeding in the last 6 months. In addition, she is experiencing occasional hot flashes. Her primary care physician had ordered a pelvic sonogram, which showed multiple uterine fibroids that were unchanged when compared to her sonogram of 2 years prior. The remainder of the patient's history and physical exam is unremarkable. What is the most appropriate next step in the management of this patient?

A. Endometrial biopsy

B. Hysterectomy

C. Combination oral contraceptives

D. Myomectomy

A Assessment of the endometrium to rule out uterine carcinoma is essential in this perimenopausal woman. Additionally, the patient is obese, which is a known risk factor for endometrial hyperplasia and carcinoma. Therefore, the best next step in the management of this patient is an endometrial biopsy. Office sampling using a Novak currette, Pipelle, or Vabra aspirator is simple, safe, and cost-effective. Office endometrial biopsies are found to be at least 95% as accurate as dilation and curettage, which requires operating room time and expense as well as risks of anesthesia.

Surgery of any kind (hysterectomy or myomectomy) is not appropriate if uterine carcinoma has not yet been ruled out. The patient may require more extensive surgery if endometrial carcinoma is suspected. Furthermore, even if an endometrial biopsy is performed and does not show atypical hyperplasia or carcinoma, surgery may not be the appropriate next step. Medical management should be attempted first if the patient is hemodynamically stable.

Combination oral contraceptive pills (OCPs) are effective in managing perimenopausal symptoms and irregular bleeding in women who are healthy nonsmokers. However, endometrial carcinoma must first be ruled out via endometrial sampling. OCPs have the added benefit of contraception in the perimenopausal woman, who is often still ovulating but does not desire pregnancy.

2 A 27-year-old obese, nulligravid woman presents with a long history of irregular vaginal bleeding. For the past 3 years her menses have been occurring every 4–7 weeks, with heavy flow. She was recently diagnosed with diabetes; otherwise, her medical history is unremarkable. On physical exam, there is evidence of facial and lower abdominal hair growth. Her pelvic exam is within normal limits. What the most likely cause of her abnormal vaginal bleeding?

A. Anovulation

B. Persistent corpus luteum

C. Cervical polyp

D. Medications

A This patient most likely has dysfunctional uterine bleeding (DUB) secondary to polycystic ovary syndrome. Polycystic ovary syndrome or chronic hyperandrogenic anovulation can cause obesity, hirsutism, insulin resistance, and menstrual disturbances. Anovulation is the predominant cause of DUB, which is defined as abnormal uterine bleeding without a demonstrable organic cause.

Occasionally, DUB can be associated with ovulation and a persistent corpus luteum. However, anovulation is a much more frequent cause. There is no evidence to suggest that this patient has a cervical polyp. No polyp was seen on pelvic exam, and cervical polyps are more commonly associated with intermenstrual and postcoital bleeding. Finally, there is no evidence that medications are the cause of her abnormal uterine bleeding. She has no history to suggest that she is taking any psychotropic, antidepressant, hormonal, or anticoagulant medications.

3 A 22-year-old woman gravida 1, para 1, presents complaining of irregular light vaginal bleeding since having an uncomplicated vaginal delivery 9 months ago. She has not yet had a normal menses and is not breastfeeding. She is taking medroxyprogesterone acetate (Depo-Provera) every 3 months for contraception. She has no other complaints. Her history and physical exam, including pelvic exam, are unremarkable. What is the most appropriate next step in the management of this patient?

A. Endometrial biopsy

B. Combination oral contraceptives

C. Intravenous estrogens

D. Observation for 3 months

D The etiology of this woman's irregular light vaginal bleeding is most likely the medroxyprogesterone acetate (Depo-Provera). Approximately 30% of women taking medroxyprogesterone will experience irregular breakthrough bleeding for the first year. About 75% of women are amenorrheic after the first year. Observing for 3 months and reassuring the patient that her light bleeding is not worrisome or abnormal is the best management for this patient. If the patient finds continued vaginal bleeding intolerable, she can be offered combination oral contraceptives, which are very effective in reducing or eliminating breakthrough bleeding.

Endometrial sampling to rule-out uterine carcinoma is usually not necessary in patients younger than 30-years of age. She has no notable risk factors for endometrial cancer. Intravenous estrogens are not necessary for this patient. She is having only light vaginal bleeding. Patients with severe endometrial atrophy causing significant hemorrhage will benefit from IV estrogens.

37

Hyperandrogenism

Tara Sosna

1 An 18-year-old nulligravid woman presents with complaints of heavy vaginal bleeding for 10 days and pelvic pain for 2 weeks. Her last menstrual period was 6 months ago. She began menses at age 13, but her periods have always been irregular, about 5 times per year. On physical exam, the patient is 63 inches tall and weighs 180 pounds. She has oily skin with mild pustular acne on her face and has dark hair growth on her chin, chest, and abdomen. Pelvic exam reveals brown, velvety discoloration of the skin on her inner thighs, a normal-sized uterus, and adnexa without masses. Laboratory evaluation reveals normal thyroid-stimulating hormone (TSH) and prolactin levels. Which of the following laboratory findings would you expect in this patient?

A. Ratio of luteinizing hormone (LH) to follicle-stimulating hormone (FSH) of less than 2

B. Elevated DHEAS level greater than 700 mg/dL

C. Elevated concentration of circulating sex hormone-binding globulin (SHBG)

D. Glucose-to-insulin ratio less than 4.5

E. Androstenedione level less than 60 ng/dL

D Hyperandrogenemic chronic anovulation syndrome (also described as polycystic ovary syndrome) is characterized by evidence of hyperandrogenism coupled with a history of 6 or fewer vaginal bleeding episodes per year. Symptoms may include hirsutism (growth of dark terminal hair on the face, chest, back, lower abdomen, and upper thighs), pustular acne, oily skin, male pattern baldness, obesity, infertility, and pelvic pain. Acanthosis nigrans is a gray-brown velvety discoloration of the skin and is a reliable indicator of the insulin resistance and hyperinsulinemia that is often associated with this syndrome. A fasting glucose-to-insulin ratio of less than 4.5 is consistent with insulin resistance.

In hyperandrogenemic chronic anovulation syndrome, an increase in the ratio of LH to FSH from 1 to greater than 2 is observed secondary to disordered regulation of hypothalamic-pituitary secretion of gonadotropin-releasing hormone. DHEAS levels are used to assess adrenal function and will be normal or mildly elevated in hyperandrogenemic chronic anovulation. The normal range is 38–338 μg/dL. Levels higher than 700 ng/dL are consistent with abnormal adrenal function, and may suggest an adrenal androgen-producing tumor if they are higher than 1,000 ng/dL. SHBG production by the liver is decreased secondary to the effect of insulin, thereby causing increases in the level of free and active testosterone. The normal serum concentration of androstenedione in women ranges from 60 to 300 ng/dL. These levels are elevated in hyperandrogenemic chronic anovulation syndrome secondary to increased secretion by theca cells in response to LH stimulation. Androstenedione produces an androgenic biologic effect when present in excess amounts.

2 A 20-year-old gravida 1, para 0010, presents with complaints of new onset of increased facial hair growth and thinning of hair in the temporal region of the scalp and the crown of her head. She reports menarche at the age of 11, with periods every 28–90 days since that time. The physical exam is significant only for male pattern baldness and facial and abdominal hirsutism. Laboratory evaluation reveals normal TSH, prolactin, FSH, and LH. Testosterone and androstenedione levels are mildly elevated, and DHEAS is normal. Morning basal 17-hydroxyprogesterone level is 585 ng/dL. What should the next step in her evaluation be?

A. Pelvic ultrasound

B. High-dose dexamethasone suppression test with measurement of blood adrenocorticotropic hormone (ACTH) levels

C. ACTH stimulation testing with synthetic ACTH

D. Measurement of morning and afternoon plasma cortisol levels

E. Measurement of 24-hour urinary free cortisol level

C The elevated morning basal 17-hydroxyprogesterone (17-OHP) level, greater than 200 ng/dL, suggests late-onset adrenal hyperplasia in this patient. The most common adrenal enzyme defect is 21-hydroxylase (21-OH). The 21-OH converts progesterone to deoxycorticosterone, or 17-OHP to deoxycortisol, and a deficiency in this enzyme causes a decrease in cortisol production. This leads to increased secretion of ACTH by the pituitary. Increased ACTH stimulation of the adrenal gland causes increased production of 17-OHP, which is in turn converted to androstenedione by the enzyme 17α-hydroxylase-17,20-desmolase. Androstenedione is then converted to testosterone by 17-ketosteroid reductase, leading to hyperandrogenic symptoms.

The next step in evaluation of this patient should be ACTH-stimulation testing with a 25 units of cortrosyn. A 17-OHP level greater than 1,200 ng/dL after 1 hour will confirm the diagnosis of late-onset adrenal hyperplasia. Choices **B**, **D**, and **E** are laboratory tests used to diagnose Cushing syndrome. Choice **A**, a pelvic ultrasound, should be used when an ovarian androgen-producing tumor is suspected.

3 A 27-year-old nulligravida presents with new-onset hirsutism that is rapidly progressing. The patient also reports recent deepening of the voice, recession of frontal hair, reduction of breast size, and increased muscle mass of her arms and legs. Physical exam reveals a palpable adnexal mass on the right side. Testosterone level is 390 ng/dL, and DHEAS level is 500 μg/dL. What is the most appropriate treatment for this patient?

A. Flutamide 250 mg/day

B. Finasteride 5 mg/day

C. Oral contraceptive pills $\times$ 6 months

D. Medroxyprogesterone acetate 10 mg/day for 10–12 days per month

E. Surgical exploration

E The palpation of an adnexal mass, testosterone levels exceeding 200 ng/dL, and symptoms of hyperandrogenism or rapid onset of virulization as seen in this patient suggest an ovarian androgen-producing tumor such as a Sertoli-Leydig cell, a granulosa-theca cell, or a Hilus cell tumor. Surgery is the treatment of choice. Depending on the type of tumor, additional treatment with chemotherapy or radiation may be required. Choices **A–D** are appropriate therapies for hyperandrogenemic chronic anovulation syndrome or idiopathic hirsutism (5–15% of all hirsute patients).

Flutamide is a nonsteroidal antiandrogen that blocks the binding of testosterone to its receptors. Finasteride inhibits type II 5-α reductase, the enzyme that catalyzes the conversion of testosterone to dihydrotestosterone in some tissues. OCPs act by diminishing circulating gonadotropin levels and increasing SHBG levels, causing lower circulating levels of androgen. Medroxyprogesterone acetate is used to produce regular withdrawal bleeding to reduce the risk of menorrhagia and endometrial hyperplasia.

Please read the following vignette to answer Questions 4 and 5.

A 28-year-old gravida 0, para 0, nulligravida presents with complaints of amenorrhea and infertility. She has been on oral contraceptive pills for 10 years, secondary to a history of dysfunctional uterine bleeding and persistent ovarian cysts. Eleven months ago, she patient discontinued the pills, but she did not have a period for 6 months. At that time her doctor gave her medroxyprogesterone acetate for 10 days to stimulate a withdrawal bleed. Since then she has had two menstrual periods, but monitoring of her basal body temperature charts demonstrates no evidence of ovulation.

---

4 Which of the following treatments should be used first in this patient who desires fertility?

A. Oral contraceptive pills plus metformin hydrochloride 500 mg TID for 6 months

B. Oral clomiphene citrate (50–100 mg) for 5 days on a monthly basis

C. Oral clomiphene citrate (50–100 mg) for 5 days plus metformin hydrochloride 500 mg TID

D. Systemic administration of gonadotropins

E. Spironolactone 100–200 mg per day for 6 months

B Ovulation induction in women with hyperandrogenemic chronic anovulation syndrome can be achieved with clomiphene citrate in about 80% of cases. Clomiphene citrate acts by blocking the binding of estrogen to its receptor in the hypothalamus and is administered orally in doses of 50–100 mg per day for 5 days on a monthly basis. Metformin may considered in a well-informed patient who is unable to ovulate using clomiphene citrate alone. Gonadotropin injections may be used to stimulate the ovary directly if clomiphene therapy is unsuccessful.

5 A patient develops a deep vein thrombosis during her pregnancy and is no longer able to use oral contraceptive pills. Postpartum, she has an intrauterine device placed for contraception, but desires treatment for hirsutism. Which of the following medications would not be effective?

A. Spironolactone

B. Danazol

C. Flutamide

D. Finasteride

B Choices **A**, **C**, and **D** are effective treatments for hirsutism. Choice **B**, Danazol, a 17α-ethinyl derivative of testosterone, is used for the treatment of endometriosis and may cause iatrogenic hirsutism.

Spironolactone, an aldosterone antagonist, is often initiated if OCPs are contraindicated or suboptimal. It inhibits DHT binding to its receptors and decreases the ovarian production and clearance testosterone. The drug is effective in 60–70% of women with hirsutism. Flutamide, a nonsteroidal antiandrogen, also blocks the binding of testosterone to its receptor and is effective in decreasing terminal hair diameter and growth. Finasteride treats hirsutism by inhibiting the type II 5α-reductase conversion of testosterone to DHT in some tissues.

38

Female Sexual Function and Dysfunction

Julie Jolin

1 A 30-year-old woman, who recently began taking a selective serotonin reuptake inhibitor (SSRI) for postpartum depression 6 months following delivery, complains of decreased desire for sexual intercourse, and anorgasmia. The most appropriate course of action is to

A. Consider sildenafil citrate to alleviate SSRI-induced sexual dysfunction

B. Change from an SSRI to bupropion hydrochloride to treat depression

C. Add bupropion to the SSRI regimen

D. Any of the above

D Postpartum depression is a serious and common complication of pregnancy, affecting 10–15% of women following deliveries. Its typical onset is in the first 3 months postpartum, but may have a more insidious onset more than 6 months after delivery. Symptoms of postpartum depression are similar to that of a major depressive disorder, including depressed mood, decreased interest or pleasure in activities, change in appetite or weight, insomnia or hypersomnia, feeling restless or slowed down, fatigue, decreased concentration, feelings of guilt or worthlessness, and suicidal ideation. Specifically, postpartum women may suffer from ambivalent or negative feelings toward the infant, and self-doubt concerning the ability to care for the child. Antidepressant medications along with psychotherapy are considered as initial treatments for major depressive episodes.

Although highly effective antidepressants such as the SSRIs are now routinely prescribed, it is important to counsel women regarding potential side effects. Nearly 60% of women taking SSRIs suffer from some form of sexual dysfunction, including decreased desire and arousal, and anorgasmia. It is postulated that this dysfunction results from increased serotonin effect and decreased dopaminergic effect on the central nervous system. All three recommendations listed above have been shown to decrease SSRI-induced sexual dysfunction.

2 You are asked by the psychiatry department to participate in a joint conference on female sexual function. Of the following models of female sexual response, the most contemporary is the

A. Masters and Johnson model

B. Basson model

C. Johnson model

D. Kaplan model

B Masters and Johnson devised the first model of female sexual response in 1966, which identified excitement, plateau, orgasm, and resolution occurring in successive phases. Kaplan revised the Masters and Johnson model in 1974 to simplify the stages into desire, arousal, and orgasm. In 2000, Basson diagrammed a model based on Kaplan's stages but included the psychosocial aspects of the female sexual response. Basson's model of female sexual response aims to depict more accurately the responsive component of women's desire and the underlying motivational forces that trigger it. The model also acknowledges the variety of arousal responses a woman may experience. Basson's stated purpose for revising the model is both to prevent diagnosing dysfunction when the response is simply different from the traditional human sex-response cycle and to more clearly define subgroups of dysfunction.

3 A 42-year-old woman complains that she has been unable to become sexually excited recently, despite strong desire for sexual contact with her partner with whom she has been involved for 10 years. She denies any pain during noncoital or coital stimulation. According to the 1998 American Foundation of Urologic Diseases Consensus Panel, her recent condition would be classified as

A. Hypoactive sexual desire
B. Sexual aversion disorder
C. Sexual arousal disorder
D. Orgasmic disorder
E. Sexual pain disorder

C In 1998, an international multidisciplinary panel established a classification system to guide research and treatment of female sexual dysfunction. The classification includes physiologic and psychogenic causes of dysfunction. Hypoactive sexual desire involves persistent or recurrent deficiency or absence of sexual fantasies and thoughts, or the absence of desire for or receptivity to sexual activity. Sexual aversion disorder is the persistent or recurrent phobic aversion to and avoidance of sexual contact. Sexual arousal disorder is the persistent or recurrent inability to attain or to maintain sufficient sexual excitement. Orgasmic disorder involves the persistent or recurrent difficulty in, delay in, or absence of attaining orgasm after sufficient sexual stimulation and arousal. Sexual pain disorders include dyspareunia, vaginismus, and noncoital sexual pain.

4 A 66-year-old woman presents for routine gynecologic care, at which time she reports being sexually active, but having problems with decreased genital sensation, and increased dyspareunia. The remainder of the history is unremarkable, with the exception of having a 20-year history of diabetes. In general, when considering a patient such as this, which of the following statements regarding postmenopausal sexual dysfunction is most accurate?

A. Serum estradiol levels below 200 pg/mL are correlated with complaints of sexual dysfunction.

B. Androgens contribute greatly to sexual desire and overall libido, but have not been shown to contribute to strength of female genital tissues.

C. Long-standing, poorly controlled diabetes mellitus may result in peripheral neuropathy, which may result in decreased sensation, or even pain, in the vagina and clitoris.

D. Selective serotonin reuptake inhibitors (SSRIs) have been shown to result in less sexual dysfunction than bupropion hydrochloride.

C Estrogens, androgens, oxytocin, and dopaminergic agonists are believed to promote the female sexual response, whereas progesterone, prolactin, and serotonin are thought to play an inhibitory role. Postmenopausal women with estradiol levels below 50 pg/mL report increased complaints of sexual dysfunction, including decreased desire, decreased sexual response, decreased genital sensation, decreased orgasm, and increased dyspareunia. While the exact physiologic and biochemical role of androgens in female sexual response is unclear, testosterone replacement has been shown to improve sexual desire, arousal, and orgasm. Furthermore, data show that androgens contribute to the structural and metabolic integrity of female genital tissues. SSRIs have been shown to cause sexual dysfunction in nearly 60% of patients, thought to be due to an increased serotonin effect and decreased dopaminergic effect in the central nervous system. Bupropion has been shown to be an effective addition to or substitute for SSRIs in treating SSRI-induced sexual dysfunction.

Whenever a woman is being assessed for sexual dysfunction, it is important to focus on medical history, current medications, and social history, which often reveal the underlying cause. A medical history includes systemic conditions such as hypertension, diabetes mellitus, depression, and multiple sclerosis, all of which predispose a patient to sexual dysfunction. Current medications may have a significantly adverse effect on libido or sexual function. Dependence on cigarettes, alcohol, or other illicit drugs, may also clearly affect sexual function.

39

Menopause

Kim Fortner

1 A 48-year-old woman visits the office complaining of mood symptoms and wants to know if she has reached the perimenopausal period. Her complete history reveals many years of endometriosis, controlled by oral contraceptives since her late 30s. In order to evaluate her menopausal status:

A. It is not possible to evaluate patients for menopause during oral contraceptive use; therefore she should have her follicle-stimulating hormone (FSH) level evaluated at least 6 weeks after discontinuance of her pills.

B. It is not possible to evaluate patients for menopause during oral contraceptive use; therefore she should have her luteinizing hormone (LH) level evaluated 6 weeks after discontinuance of her pills.

C. It is possible to evaluate patients for menopause by measuring serum FSH twice during the active pill weeks.

D. It is possible to evaluate patients for menopause by measuring FSH late in the pill-free week.

D This question pertains to perimenopause; the period of perimenopause is defined as lasting from before menopause to up to 1 year after the onset of menopause. Recall that when doubt exists about the diagnosis of menopause, other causes of amenorrhea must be ruled out. Laboratory studies should include a pregnancy test, prolactin, and an FSH level. Women on oral contraceptives can be evaluated while still continuing their pill use. A serum FSH level may be measured late in the pill-free week. When the serum FSH level is persistently elevated during the pill-free week, the patient is likely menopausal. At this time, she can be switched to hormone replacement therapy (HRT), after she has been counseled extensively regarding the risks and benefits.

2 A 69-year-old patient comes to your office complaining of back pains. Her husband says she is "shrinking." Her history is significant for menopause at age 49, managed initially on hormone replacement therapy until she was diagnosed with breast cancer. She has a history of breast cancer and hepatitis. She is a thin Caucasian female with a normal physical examination including breast and pelvic exams. The best therapy for her following a complete workup will most likely be

A. Oral hormone replacement therapy (HRT)

B. Oral calcitonin

C. Oral raloxifene

D. Transdermal clonidine

C This patient most likely has osteoporosis, defined as a condition of decreased bone mass and deterioration of bone architecture with resulting skeletal fractures. Deficiency of estrogen causes an increased rate of bone remodeling. Risk factors for osteoporosis include Caucasian race, advancing age, estrogen deficiency, etc. (Table 39-2 of the *Johns Hopkins Manual of Gynecology and Obstetrics*). The first-line therapy is identification and modification of risk factors. Further recommendations include taking calcium and vitamin D, as well as participating in routine weight-bearing exercise.

The diagnosis of osteoporosis is made by determination of bone mineral density (BMD). If dual-energy X-ray absorptiometry (DEXA) is performed and yields a T-score of −1.0 or below, then the patient has osteopenia; with a T-score of −2.5 or below, the diagnosis is osteoporosis.

Prior to the Women's Health Initiative (WHI) study, no large prospective studies had shown that estrogen decreases fractures; however, the unadjusted risk of hip fracture revealed a reduced fracture rate on HRT. This patient, however, is not a candidate for HRT, given that she is a breast cancer survivor. The relationship between breast cancer and HRT is still an area of active research.

Oral calcitonin is degraded by stomach acid. Intranasal calcitonin, like Miacalcin, has been used effectively for the treatment of osteoporosis. Calcitonin, which inhibits bone resorption by decreasing osteoclastic activity, will not necessarily be the best first-line agent for this patient.

Alternative therapies such as selective estrogen receptor modulators can be employed when there is a contraindication to HRT. Raloxifene has estrogen agonist properties in bone and the cardiovascular system, but antiestrogen effects in breast and uterus. A large controlled trial showed that BMD increased 2.4% for L-spine and 2.0% for hip, LDL decreased with no difference in endometrial thickness. The MORE study showed that in women taking raloxifene, 5.4–6.6% had new vertebral fractures, versus 10.1% in women taking placebo. There was, however, an increased incidence of thromboembolic disease, hot flashes, influenza-like symptoms, and leg cramps.

Transdermal clonidine has been shown to be useful in the treatment of hot flashes, not osteoporosis.

3 A 69-year-old patient comes to your office complaining of worsening heartburn despite use of antiacids, increasing abdominal pain between meals, and diarrhea. Which of the following medications is she likely taking?

A. Clonidine

B. Risedronate

C. Raloxifene

D. Calcitonin

B This patient is likely experiencing the side effects of a bisphosphonate. Bisphosphonates are approved for the treatment and prevention of osteoporosis. They help to inhibit bone resorption and are shown to progressively increase bone mass at hip and spine. The main difficulty with these medications is their absorption and effect on the gastrointestinal tract. They cause heartburn, esophagitis, abdominal pain, and diarrhea. It is recommended that these medications be taken in the morning after an overnight fast, sitting straight up, with consumption of adequate amounts of water.

Clonidine is often used in the treatment of hot flashes. The side effects include those that pertain to hypotension: lightheadedness or dizziness on standing.

Raloxifene is a selective estrogen receptor modulator (SERM) that has been approved for use in treatment and prevention of osteoporosis. SERMs have an agonistic effect on bone and the cardiovascular system and an antagonistic effect on breast and uterus. Use of SERMs correlates with increases in BMD compared to patients taking placebo. The side effects include hot flashes and leg cramps. There is also an increased risk of thromboembolic events.

Calcitonin is a peptide hormone that inhibits bone resorption by decreasing osteoclastic activity. Parenteral administration is required due to degradation of the peptide when taken orally. Side effects include nausea and flushing. Rhinitis and epistaxis may occur with Miacalcin, an intranasal form of calcitonin.

4 A 46-year-old gravida 2, para 2, comes to the office complaining of heavy vaginal bleeding. She reports she is having her period every 15 days, passing clots, with heavier bleeding than usual. Review of systems reveals occasional hot flashes, but no other symptoms or positive findings. After an endometrial biopsy and evaluation to rule out neoplasm, she would benefit most from initiation of:

A. Depo-Provera

B. Oral contraceptive pills (OCPs)

C. Clonidine

D. Estrogen replacement therapy

B The patient has anovulatory bleeding. The changing hormones of the perimenopausal period can lead to anovulatory bleeding and complaints of irregular, heavy bleeding. If the bleeding occurs more frequently than every 21 days, lasts longer than 8 days, and is very heavy, a workup should be undertaken to rule out neoplasm.

Control of the perimenopausal vaginal bleeding unrelated to neoplasm can be attained with oral contraceptives pills. Oral contraceptive pills will stabilize the endometrium, decrease vasomotor symptoms, and establish more regular menses during the perimenopausal period. In addition, the pills can provide contraception and lead to increased bone mineral density. A lower-dose pill with 20 μg of estrogen has equal efficacy and fewer side effects than a 30- or 35-μg pill. A patient can then be transitioned to HRT or taken off the OCPs once she is in her mid-50s or once her FSH level is higher than 20 IU/mL on day 6 or 7 of the pill-free week.

5 Reported benefits of hormone replacement therapy include all of the following *except:*

A. Protection from colon cancer

B. Prevention of osteoporosis

C. Treatment of osteoporosis

D. Prevention of breast cancer

E. Prevention of vaginal atrophy

D HRT has been associated with an increase in a woman's risk of developing breast cancer and has been the subject of much investigation. The Collaborative Group of Hormonal Factors in Breast Cancer found that the risk of breast cancer in current users and women who had recently stopped HRT (1–4 years ago) was 1.023 highor per year of use. In women taking HRT for more than 5 years, the relative risk was 1.35.

Hormone replacement therapy has come under scrutiny since the Women's Health Initiative (WHI), with the benefits and risks being reexamined. Studies still support that HRT helps prevent and treat osteoporosis, as evidenced by WHI data showing a reduced rate of hip and vertebral fractures in women using HRT. In addition, HRT is used in the treatment of osteoporosis. The WHI also supported that the risk of colorectal cancer was lower in women taking HRT, consistent with prior studies. Lastly, estrogen, whether taken orally, transdermal, or vaginally, does treat vaginal atrophy.

40

Benign Vulvar Lesions

Carolyn Alexander

Please read the following vignette to answer Questions 1 and 2.

An 81-year-old woman, gravida 0, para 0, presents to your clinic complaining of vulvar itching. Her past medical history is significant for hypertention, atrial fibrillation, and gastroesophageal reflux. Her last Pap smear was over 20 years ago. Her past surgical history includes a supracervical hysterectomy for symptomatic fibroids. She is currently not taking hormone replacement therapy. She stopped smoking 20 years ago. She has an otherwise negative review of systems.

---

1 Which of the following is the least likely cause of her pruritic?

A. Vulvar intraepithelial lesion (VIN)
B. Candidal vaginitis
C. Atrophic vulvitis
D. Molluscum contagiosum
E. Lichen sclerosis

D Molluscum contagiosum is typically an asymptomatic superficial infection with viral replication limited to the epidermis. Characteristic morphology includes umbilicated papules as well as inflammation, irritation, and secondary infection. Confirmation of the diagnosis can be made by microscopic evaluation of the

TABLE 40.1	Causes of Vulvar Pruritus
Infections	
Candida	
Trichomonas	
Bacterial vaginosis	
Hidradenitis suppurativa	
Herpes simplex	
Human papillomavirus	
Dermatophytes	
Scabies	
Dermatoses	
Lichen sclerosis	
Lichen simplex chronicus	
Lichen planus (erosive vaginitis)	
Psoriasis	
Seborrheic dermatitis	
Low Estrogen States: Atrophic Vaginitis	
Postpartum	
Postmenopausal	
Premalignant/Malignant Conditions	
Vulvar intraepithelial neoplasia	
Squamous cell carcinoma	
Adenocarcinoma	
Irritants	
Contact dermatitis	

caseous material obtained from curetting of the lesion. Homogeneous inclusion bodies within the keratinocytes, known as molluscum bodies (i.e., Henderson-Paterson bodies), are pathognomonic for this disease. These bodies form as a result of virally induced transformation within the infected keratinocytes.

Choice **A** is incorrect because patients with VIN may present with itching, vulvar irritation, dyspareunia, labial erythema, or swelling. Currently, VIN is defined histologically as a disorientation of epithelial architecture that is limited by the basement membrane, with no extension to the underlying dermis. VIN 1 is mild dysplasia, VIN 2 is moderate dysplasia, and VIN 3 is severe dysplasia/carcinoma *in situ.*

Choice **B** is incorrect because the predominant symptom of candidal vaginitis is vulvar pruritis. The classic vaginal discharge is white, curdlike, and without an odor. Choice **C** is incorrect because atrophic vulvitis is associated with pruritis. Withdrawal of estradiol during menopause results in thinning of the vaginal and vulvar epithelial layers, a reduction in overall mitotic activity, hypoestrogenic changes in the vaginal and urethral epithelium, and a decrease in tissue vascularity. Choice **E** is incorrect because lichen sclerosis is associated with vulvar pruritis. The lesions are typically scattered patches of porcelain white, atrophic, indurated plaques, most commonly on the vulva. Fissures of the skin may develop in the posterior fourchette, as well as large ulcers because of intense scratching.

2 The physical examination reveals multiple white plaques on the labia minora. The most important next step in evaluation of this woman's disorder is

A. Papanicolaou (Pap) smear
B. Colposcopy
C. Punch biopsy
D. Apply podophyllin
E. Culture the lesion

C Liberal use of punch biopsy is recommended to make an accurate diagnosis of any lesion on the vulva, in order to rule out invasive disease. Making sure the patient is up to date on her Pap smear is important, but a biopsy of this lesion is critical. Application of acetic acid with colposcopic magnification may be helpful, but several minutes are required for the keratinized squamous epithelium to take up the solution. Abnormal vessel patterns are not commonly seen, owing to the keratinization of vulvar skin. Toluidine blue staining may be helpful but lacks sensitivity or specificity. Application of podophyllin resin is used for patients with genital warts and would not be used in this patient. Furthermore, culturing these white plaques on the vulva is not necessary.

3 Match the following with their description:

A. Lentigo simplex	**1.** Involves genital ulcers, which are small and deep
B. Papillary hidradenomas	**2.** Occurs along the milk line, especially on the labia majora

C. Molluscum contagiosum

D. Beçhet's syndrome

E. Vitiligo

3. The most common hyperpigmented lesion of the vulva

4. An inherited disorder in which melanocytes are lost, frequently from the vulva

5. A poxvirus leading to multiple, umbilicated papules filled with waxy material

1—D Beçhet's syndrome is a chronic, relapsing inflammatory disease characterized by recurrent oral, genital, and ocular aphthae. It is considered to be a type of multisystem vasculitis. Genital lesions occur in about 75% of patients with Beçhet's disease.

2—B Papillary hidradenomas occur along the milk line and present as firm, encapsulated nodules that can measure up to 2 cm in greatest dimension. The most frequent location is on the labia majora or in the interlabial folds.

3—A Lentigo simplex usually arises in childhood. It is most common hyperpigmented lesion of the vulva. The lesions are usually less than 6 mm, sharply demarcated, uniformly pigmented. Clinically, they may be indistinguishable from a junctional nevus.

4—E Vitiligo is thought to involve an autoimmune process directed against melanocytes. The depigmentation has a predilection for acral areas and around body orifices. The course is slowly progressive. A skin biopsy is necessary to differentiate it from other disorders.

5—C Molluscum contagiosum is a benign viral skin infection caused by a DNA-containing pox virus. Characteristic molluscum lesions are 2–5 mm in size, firm umbilicated papules filled with waxy material. They are found on the epidermal surfaces of the extremities, trunk, or genital areas, including the lower abdomen, pubic area, and inner thighs. These papules appear 2–7 weeks after contact and usually occur in crops. They often resolve spontaneously. The typical course of the disease is 6–9 months.

41

Vulvar and Vaginal Cancer

Carolyn Alexander

1 Which type of vaginal malignancy is associated with diethylstilbestrol (DES) exposure?

A. Squamous cell carcinoma
B. Leiomyosarcoma
C. Melanoma
D. Clear cell adenocarcinoma

D During the 1940s, DES treatment was used during pregnancy to prevent premature delivery and threatened abortions. In 1971, Herbst et al. described an increased risk for clear cell adenocarcinoma of the vagina in young women with *in utero* exposure to DES. Susequently, the use of estrogens for treatment of pregnancy complications in the United States was prohibited by the U.S. Food and Drug Administration. In the United States, it is estimated that approximately 3 million pregnant women were treated with DES.

2 Which of the following is the most frequent location of carcinoma in patients with DES exposure *in utero*?

A. Upper one-third of the vagina
B. Lower one-third of the vagina

C. Anterior fornix of vagina

D. Posterior fornix of vagina

A Clear cell carcinomas related to DES exposure may occur anywhere on the vagina or cervix, but most have been documented in the upper part of the vagina, particularly on the anterior wall. Adenosis is commonly seen with clear cell adenocarcinomas. Adenosis appears granular and red, and is also typically encountered on the upper anterior vaginal wall. This site is frequently hidden by the speculum blade; therefore, careful inspection of all vaginal surfaces is critical during pelvic examination. The speculum should be rotated so that anterior or posterior wall lesions are not overlooked. Routine cytologic Pap smear of the vagina should be continued even for patients who have previously undergone hysterectomy. Bimanual pelvic and rectal examinations are integral elements in the clinical evaluation of patients with a history of DES exposure, because the lesions may also be submucosal.

3 Which of the following is contraindicated in the treatment plan for verrucous carcinoma of the vulva?

A. Primary chemotherapy

B. Radical local excision

C. Radiation

D. Regional lymphadenectomy

C Verrucous carcinoma is a variant of squamous cell cancer. It presents as a large cauliflower-like, condylomatous lesion. Multiple biopsies are needed to establish the correct diagnosis. Although it is typically invasive, it rarely metastasizes. Treatment with wide local excision is recommended. Anaplastic transformation with subsequent regional and distant metastasis has been reported with radiation therapy.

Please read the following vignette to answer Questions 4–7.
A 71-year-old gravida 3, para 3003, presents with clinic complaints of vulvar pruritis for 3 years. On physical examination,

the patient has a sharply demarcated, red lesion with slightly raised edges and islands of white epithelium on the right labium majus.

---

4 What is the best first step in evaluation?

A. Observation

B. Colposcopic examination

C. Biopsy

D. Wide local excision

C Paget's disease of the vulva is a rare intraepithelial lesion that is typically a well-demarcated erythematous eczematoid lesion with irregular borders (Figure 41.1). It has hyperemic areas with a superficial white coating. Any vulvar lesion discovered by a physical examination should be biopsied to rule out a neoplasm. Biopsy of the lesion reveals the characteristic large eosinophilic Paget

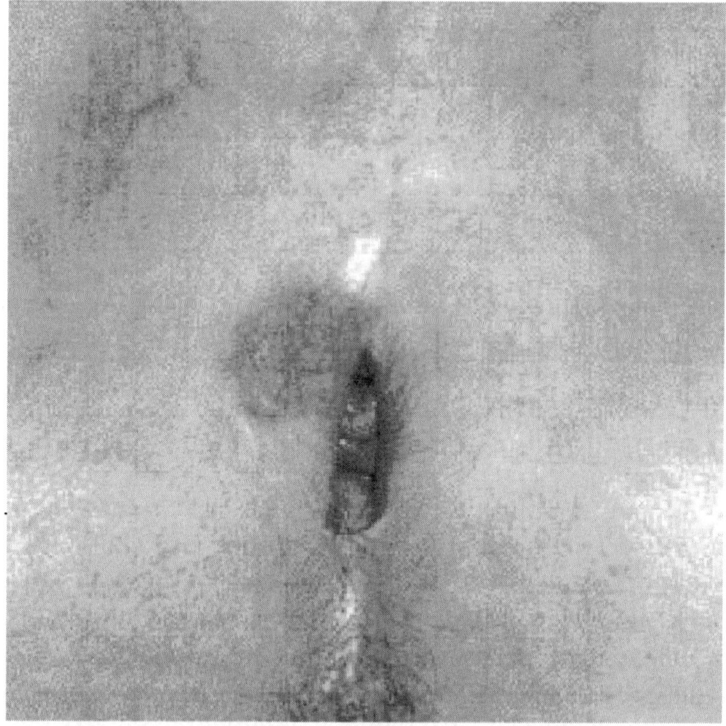

FIGURE 41.1 Image of a vulvar lesion representing Paget's disease.

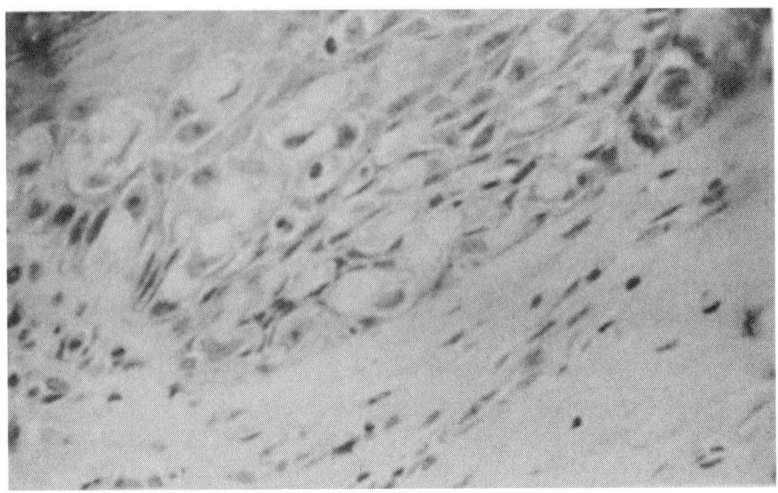

FIGURE 41.2 Histiologic image of Paget's disease of the vulva.

cells in the basal layer of the epithelium, spread within the dermis, or around dermal appendages (Figure 41.2). Attention should be given to the size and location of the lesion. When evaluating a vulvar lesion, it is important to assess the presence or absence of groin lymphadenopathy. Seventy percent of vulvar cancers occur in the labia, and 15–20% include the clitoris or the perineal body. In approximately 5% of cases, multifocal and noncontiguous lesions occur.

5 Colposcopic evaluation demonstrated a unilateral vulvar lesion, but the cervix and vagina were normal. If a biopsy reveals Paget's disease limited to the epithelium, which of the following is the best treatment plan?

A. Close observation

B. Wide local excision

C. Partial vulvectomy

D. Radical excision and inguinal lymphadenectomy

B When the biopsy reveals Paget's disease limited to the epithelium, a wide local excision for small lesions produces excellent results. If no local or distant primary malignancy is uncovered, it is important to remove the full thickness of the vulvar skin to the adipose layer, as it may have a subclinical malignancy. A conservative approach with a 1-cm margin appears to be most appropriate. Reexcision may be required for recurrence in the future.

6 If a biopsy reveals Paget's disease with an underlying adenocarcinoma invading the upper urethra, which of the following is the proper FIGO stage?

A. Stage II
B. Stage III
C. Stage IVA
D. Stage IVB

C Paget's disease with an underlying adenocarcinoma invading the upper urethra is considered stage IVA. The International Federation of Gynecology and Obstetrics (FIGO) staging system for vulvar cancer is given in Table 41.1.

7 Which of the following is the appropriate treatment for the above lesion?

A. Wide local excision
B. Partial vulvectomy

TABLE 41.1 **Staging for Vulvar Cancer**

Stage	Description
0	Carcinoma *in situ*
I	Tumor confined to vulva or perineum; lesion < 2 cm; no palpable nodes
II	Tumor confined to vulva or perineum; lesion > 2 cm; no palpable nodes
III	Tumor of any size extending to lower urethra, vagina, or anus and/or unilateral nodal metastasis
IVA	Tumor invading upper urethra, bladder, rectal mucosa, or pelvic bone, with or without regional nodal metastasis
IVB	Distant metastasis to any site, including pelvic lymph nodes

C. Radical excision

D. Radical excision and regional inguinal lymphadenectomy

D Paget's disease may extend well beyond the gross lesion, resulting in positive surgical margins. Underlying adenocarinomas may be clinically apparent. As a result, laser therapy is inadequate treatment. Paget's disease with an underlying adenocarcinoma invading the upper urethra requires radical excision and regional inguinal lymphadenectomy.

42

Cervical Intraepithelial Neoplasia

Julie Huh

1 Which of the following statements is true?

A. Worldwide, cervical cancer is not considered an important cause of cancer death in women.

B. Human papilloma virus (HPV) infection is uncommon in women.

C. Risk factors for cervical intraepithelial neoplasia (CIN) include HPV infection, multiple sexual partners, intercourse at an early age, immunocompromise, other sexually transmitted diseases, and cigarette smoking.

D. Nearly all CIN lesions arise in the endocervix.

C Risk factors for CIN include HPV infection, multiple sexual partners, intercourse at an early age, immunocompromise, other sexually transmitted diseases, and cigarette smoking. Worldwide, cervical cancer is the second-leading cause of cancer death in women. HPV infection is common among women, and more than 70% of women will have had an infection by the end of their sexual experience. Nearly all CIN lesions arise in the transformation zone, which is the area of glandular epithelium that undergoes a process of squamous metaplasia.

2 Which of the following statements regarding the progression of CIN is true?

A. Approximately 90% of CIN I lesions regress spontaneously.

B. Less than 5% of CIN I lesions progress to CIN III.

C. 0.1% of lesions may ultimately progress to invasive cancer.

D. Persistent positive test results for oncogenic HPV types may indicate a significant risk for the development of high-grade squamous intraepithelial lesion (HSIL) and cancer.

D Persistent positive test results for oncogenic HPV types may indicate a significant risk for the development of HSIL and cancer. Approximately 60% of CIN I lesions regress spontaneously. Ten percent of CIN I lesions progress to CIN III, and 1% may ultimately progress to invasive cancer.

3 Which of the following is recommended management of atypical glandular cells (AGC) identified on Pap smears?

A. Vaginal colposcopy and endocervical curettage (ECC)

B. Repeat Pap smear every 4–6 months until four normal Pap smear results are obtained

C. Cervical conization

D. Colposcopy with endometrial biopsy if the patient is over age 35

D Women with atypical glandular cells have a significantly greater risk of developing cervical neoplasia than women with atypical squamous cells or LSIL. Therefore, they should be evaluated by colposcopy. If the patient is over age 35 or if the the Pap smear reveals atypical endometrial cells, then endometrial sampling is warranted because of the increased risk of endometrial hyperplasia or carcinoma.

43

Cervical Cancer

Muna Tahlak

1 A 30-year-old woman who tests positive for the human immunodeficiency virus (HIV) is diagnosed with squamous cell carcinoma of the cervix, stage 1B. Aside from stage of the cancer, what is her most important prognostic factor?

A. Treatment with surgery rather than radiotherapy

B. Degree of tumor differentiation

C. HIV status

D. Human papillomavirus (HPV) infection

E. Age at diagnosis

C Cervical cancer is the most common malignancy among women with AIDS. Invasive cervical cancer is almost twice as common in HIV-infected women than in the general population. Immunocompromised women, especially those with a CD4 cell count less than 500 cells/μL, demonstrate more rapid progression from preinvasive to invasive lesions. Patients who test positive for HIV infection appear to present with invasive cervical cancer earlier than patients who test negative for the virus, and with more advanced disease at the time of diagnosis. Although stage of disease at the time of diagnosis remains the most important prognostic factor relating to survival, HIV status appears to have the next most significant influence. In one study of 28 women with all stages of cervical cancer who were HIV-positive, 88% of those followed for at least 1 year had recurrence of disease.

Patients with clinically staged FIGO stage 1B cervical cancer with AIDS have similar survival rates when either radical surgery or radiation therapy is used for primary treatment. Tumor differentiation is not a prognostic indicator in patients with squamous cell cancer of the cervix. HPV infection plays a significant role in the etiology of cervical neoplasia. HPV DNA (predominantly of types 16, 18, and 31) has been isolated from 80–100% of cervical carcinomas. Some studies have shown that younger patients (younger than 40 years) have a worse prognosis. Other studies have failed to identify any prognostic effect of age.

2 A 25-year-old gravida 3, para 2012, presented to your clinic for an annual gynecologic visit. She became sexually active at age 15 and had a series of sexual partners. She has had the same partner since age 20, and her last Pap smear 3 years ago was normal. Of the following, the factor in this patient's history that is most pertinent to her risk for cervical cancer is

A. Number of sexual partners

B. Sexual history of her male partner

C. Smoking

D. Race

E. HPV status

E Infection with HPV is now regarded as the major predictor of cervical cancer risk, with the association meeting all established criteria for epidemiologic causality. Human papillomaviruses are double-stranded DNA viruses of approximately 8,000 base pairs. There are over 80 types of HPV known. HPV 2 and 4 cause mainly common skin warts, while types 6 and 11 are the most common agents of venereal warts (condyloma accuminatum) and laryngeal polyps. A large international study of 1,000 biopsy specimens of invasive cancer from 22 countries found HPV DNA in 93% of specimens, half of which were of HPV type 16. HPV 18 accounted for an additional 10–15% and was particularly common in cervical adenocarcinomas (40–50%).

Cervical cancer risk is directly proportional to the number of lifetime sexual partners. The most direct evidence for a male factor derives from studies in which the sexual histories of husbands of cervical cancer patients have been compared with those of control husbands. In all of these studies, the husbands of cancer patients reported significantly more sexual partners than husbands of the controls.

In recent years, cigarette smoking has been considered a significant risk for cervical cancer. In most studies, not adjusted for HPV, the excess risks for smokers have been around twofold, with the highest risk generally observed for long-term or high-intensity smokers. Smoking effects appear to be restricted to squamous cell tumors, with no relationship observed for the rarer occurrences of adenocarcinoma or adenosquamous cancer.

The incidence of cervical cancer continues to rise with age among African-Americans, but among Caucasians it plateaus after 40 years of age. This presumably reflects the influence of cytologic screening. The incidence of cervical cancer is also approximately two times higher for Hispanics and even higher for Native Americans, but Asian groups experience rates similar to those of whites. When adjustment is made for socioeconomic differences, the excess risk of cervical cancer among African-Americans is substantially reduced, from more than 70% to less than 30%.

3 A 46-year-old woman presents with postcoital bleeding. On examination, she has a large fungating cervical lesion, 6 cm in diameter, with no obvious parametrial extension. Cervical biopsy demonstrates moderately differentiated squamous cell carcinoma with lymphovascular invasion. Chest X-ray shows no evidence of disease, and computed tomography scan shows no evidence of lymphadenopathy or liver disease. The recommended therapy for her is

A. Whole abdominal radiation therapy

B. Pelvic radiation therapy followed by brachytherapy

C. Cisplatin chemotherapy concurrent with pelvic radiation and brachytherapy followed in 6 weeks by extrafascial hysterectomy

D. Radical abdominal hysterectomy followed by pelvic radiation therapy

E. Radical trachelectomy

C Based on clinical staging system, this patient has stage 1B2 squamous cell carcinoma. Management of patients with bulky disease should be individualized. Surgical resection and primary radiotherapy meet with equally unpredictable outcomes for the bulky, barrel-shaped, FIGO stage 1B2 cervical lesions. Although hysterectomy after radiotherapy may reduce the risk of local recurrence, the Gynecologic Oncology Group (GOG) showed that it did not affect overall survival. Between 1992 and 1997, 369 patients with FIGO stage 1B2 lesions were treated under GOG protocol 123. All patients underwent external pelvic radiotherapy (4,500 cGy) as well as intracavitary treatments. They were randomized to receive either weekly IV cisplatin with radiotherapy or the radiotherapy alone. Following either treatment regimen, an extrafascial hysterectomy was performed within 3–6 weeks. Residual disease was found in 41% of patients treated with chemoradiation, compared with 52% of those treated with radiation alone ($p = 0.04$). The 3-year survival rate for patients who received chemoradiation was 83%, compared with 74% for those who received radiation alone ($p = 0.008$).

Five randomized controlled trials, which cumulatively involved 1,912 patients with cervical cancer, found that platinum-based chemotherapy, when given concurrently with radiation therapy, prolonged survival in women with locally advanced cervical cancer, stages 1B–IVA.

4 A 31-year-old woman, gravida 1, para 1, presents with an abnormal Pap test result. A colposcopy directed biopsy is suspicious for invasive cancer. A cold-knife conization is performed. The final pathology reveals a residual site of invasion that is 5 mm in depth and 4 mm wide, with no lymphovascular space involvement and negative margins. Of the following, the best next step is

A. Follow-up Pap smear

B. Simple hysterectomy

C. Chemoradiatiom

D. Brachytherapy

E. Modified class II radical hysterectomy with bilateral pelvic lymphadenectomy

E This patient has FIGO stage 1A2 cervical cancer. Microinvasive carcinoma with stromal invasion of 3.1–5.0 mm is associated with positive pelvic lymph nodes in 3.9–8.2% of cases. The preferred treatment of these lesions is modified radical (class II) hysterectomy with pelvic lymphadenectomy. Despite the fact that her margins of resection were negative, simply to follow the Pap smear result is not the recommended clinical approach because of the risk of metastasis. Likewise, simple hysterectomy would place the parametrial and lymph node regions at risk. Chemoradiation is based on the theory of synergistic cell kill—the therapeutic effect of two treatment modalities used in combination is greater than if the effects of the two modalities individually were simply added together. It is used for stage IIB through stage IVA cervical cancer and the bulky stage 1B disease. Brachytherapy would not be the treatment of choice for a 31-year-old woman, because radiation therapy produces persistent vaginal fibrosis and atrophy, with loss of both vaginal caliber and length.

5 A 27-year-old para 0 is undergoing fertility workup. On physical examination she had a 3-cm cervical mass on the posterior lip of her cervix with no obvious parametrial involvment. A biopsy of the lesion confirmed a well-differentiated squamous cell carcimona with lymphovascular space involvment. Abdominal computed tomography showed enlarged right pelvic lymph nodes. Baseline laboratory studies revealed a serum hemoglobin of 12.5 mg/dL, normal liver function test, and elevated serum creatinine levels. Her absolute contraindication for a radical trachelectomy is

A. Size of tumor

B. Lymphovascular space involvement

C. Pelvic lymph node involvement

D. Primary infertility

E. Elevated serum creatinine level

C While the mean age at which cervical cancer is diagnosed is 51 years, approximately 10–15% of women will develop cervical cancer earlier in their reproductive years. In 1987, the French gynecologist Dargent began performing radical trachelectomy in concert with laparoscopic pelvic lymphadenectomy. Although the potential benefit—preservation of fertility—is profound, the percentage of patients with cervical cancer who are candidates for radical trachelectomy is relatively small. The indications are the presence of an invasive cervical cancer (stage IA2, IB1, or IIA), the desire for future childbearing, no involvement of upper endocervical canal, and no evidence of metastasis on preoperative chest radiography and physical exam. Lesions that are 2 cm or smaller are ideal for resection. Although masses up to 3 cm can be resected, the recurrence rate is higher. Further, the absence of lymph vascular space involvement is preferred, but its presence is not an absolute contraindication.

6 A 25-year-old woman, gravida 2, para 1, underwent a cone biopsy at 23 weeks' gestation for a high-grade squamous intraepithelial lesion on her Pap smear. Final pathology reveals a 2-mm depth of invasion without lymphovascular invasion. The margins of the cone biopsy are negative. This was a planned pregnancy, and the patient would like to continue this pregnancy if possible. The best management is

A. Vaginal delivery at term
B. Cesarean delivery at term
C. Vaginal delivery at fetal lung maturity
D. Cesarean delivery at fetal lung maturity
E. Immediate hysterectomy

A This patient has an early microinvasive cervical cancer, stage IA1. Traditionally, vaginal delivery of pregnant cervical cancer patients has been avoided because of the theoretical potential for dissemination of tumor cells during cervical dilatation. However, overall survival after vaginal delivery (52.9%) is not significantly different from that after abdominal delivery (46.1%). Patients with less than 3 mm of invasion and no lymph vascular space involvement may be followed to term and delivered vaginally. The route of delivery should be determined by obstetric indications. There are no indications for an earlier delivery based on the cervical pathology. An immediate hysterectomy is not indicated, because she wishes to continue the pregnancy.

44

Cancer of the Uterine Corpus

Ruchi Garg

Please read the following vignette to answer Questions 1–5.
A 62-year-old African-American woman presents to your clinic for vaginal bleeding. She has been postmenopausal for 10 years and has not taken hormone replacement therapy. She has a history of cervical cancer, for which she received a "2-day in-hospital treatment" 40 years ago.

1 At this point the most concerning disease at the top of your differential is

A. Ovarian cancer
B. Uterine carcinosarcoma
C. Cervical cancer
D. Postmenopausal vaginal atrophy

B Uterine sarcomas are a group of tumors that contain malignant mesodermal elements. They comprise 3–5% of uterine malignancies and generally have a poor prognosis. The most common are carcinosarcomas (50%), followed by leiomyosarcomas (30%) and endometrial stromal sarcomas (15%). The median age of diagnosis of uterine carcinosarcoma (CS) is 62 years. There is some evidence to suggest that CS is three times more common in African-American women than in Caucasian women. Up to 10% of patients with CS have a history of radiation therapy, as suggested in this case where the patient was treated for cervical cancer with a 2-day in-hospital treatment. Furthermore, patients with CS most frequently present with postmenopausal bleeding.

2 Upon obtaining further history, you determine several risk factors that are concerning for endometrial malignancy. Risk factors for endometrial cancer include all of the following *except*:

A. Hypertension

B. Obesity

C. Nulliparity

D. Tobacco abuse

E. Diabetes

D The risk factors for endometrial adenocarcinoma include nulliparity, obesity, and diabetes. Hypertension is also associated with obesity and diabetes, hence has been suggested as a relative risk factor. Unlike other malignancies, tobacco abuse appears to have a protective effect on cancer of the endometrium.

3 All of the following characteristics on physical examination would support your suspicion of uterine malignancy *except*:

A. Height 5 ft, 10 in, weight 130 lbs

B. Uterus measuring approximately 14 weeks

C. Protruding polyp from the cervical os

D. Abnormal vaginal discharge intermixed with old blood

A Obesity is a well-known risk factor for uterine cancer because of the effects of estrogens (coverted by peripheral conversion of androgens) on the endometrium. As mentioned above, obesity is a risk factor for CS. Half of the affected women are found to have a polypoid mass, which often protrudes through the cervical os. Biopsy results usually confirm the diagnosis. Many patients with CS have pelvic pain or abnormal discharge.

4 The biopsy of the protruding polyp revealed uterine carcinosarcoma. All of the following diagnostic techniques have been validated for use in a patient who presents with symptoms suspicious for a uterine malignancy *except*:

A. Endometrial biopsy
B. Endovaginal ultrasonography
C. Hysteroscopy
D. Dilation and curettage
E. Computerized tomography (CT) scan

E When a patient presents with symptoms such as those mentioned above, several diagnostic options are available. Endometrial biopsy using a pipelle or curette device has high sensitivity and specificity in detecting endometrial cancer and is generally well tolerated as an office procedure. The false-negative rate is less than 10%. Endovaginal ultrasonography is useful for patients in whom an office endometrial biopsy is not feasible or is declined. Studies have demonstrated no documented cases of endometrial neoplasia in postmenopausal women with an endometrial stripe of less than 5 mm; conversely, an endometrial stripe of more than 10 mm is associated with 10–20% incidence of endometrial hyperplasia or malignancy. Therefore, patients with an endometrial stripe of larger than 5 mm should undergo sampling. Hysteroscopy enables direct visualization of the uterine cavity and lining. However, it has been demonstrated that hysteroscopic procedures may lead to increased incidence of malignant cells in peritoneal cytologic specimens at the time of surgical staging, which can up-stage the patient's disease. Dilation and curettage provides the most thorough screen for endomotrial neoplasia. CT scans can demonstrate the extent of disease, but cannot be used as diagnostic tools for the origin of cancer.

5 Which of the following are *not* true about this patient's disease?

A. Chemotherapy with ifosfamide and cisplatin has been shown to be as effective as surgical management.
B. Surgery is the only proven effective treatment total abdominal hysterectomy-bilateral salpingo-oopherectomy (TAH-BSO, peritoneal washings, tumor resection).

C. Radiation or chemotherapy or both, depending on the extent of the disease, may follow surgery.

D. Five-year survival rate for the disease within the uterus is 50%, versus 20% extrauterine.

A Surgery is the only proven effective treatment option to date for uterine sarcomas. Patients should be managed by exploratory laparotomy, TAH-BSO, peritoneal washings, and a complete tumor resection. Surgical staging, including omentectomy and lymph node sampling, offers prognostic information but has not been shown to affect survival. However, surgical staging may influence postoperative decisions regarding the appropriate follow-up and adjuvant therapy. For patients with stage I or II CS, the most effective adjuvant therapy remains controversial. Initial trial analysis suggests that adjuvant chemotherapy is warranted when compared to whole abdominal and pelvic radiation therapy as an alternative. The 5-year survival rate for CS is 50% for stage I disease and only 20% when extrauterine disease is identified.

Please read the following vignette to answer Questions 6–9. A 64-year-old woman has a history of endometrial cancer. Two years after her initial surgery, she presents to her gynecologist-oncologist with possible recurrent disease.

---

6 The most likely histology of the endometrial cancer is

A. Uterine papillary serous carcinoma

B. Endometrioid

C. Clear cell

D. Pure squamous

E. Undifferentiated

B Endometrioid is the most common type of endometrial cancer, comprising 80% of endometrial cancers, the majority of which are well-differentiated (grade 1) lesions. It is the degree of architectural distortion and cytologic atypia that distinguishes endometrioid carcinoma from its precursor lesion, complex atypical hyperplasia.

7 The pathology report states that the patient has endometrioid cancer with stage IIA, grade 2 disease. What does that mean to you as a clinician?

A. The cancer is invading her bladder.

B. There was over 50% of the tumor with solid growth pattern.

C. The disease is limited to endocervix with 6–50% of solid growth pattern.

D. She has a 60% chance of recurrence of her disease.

C Uterine cancer is surgically staged. The disease is limited to endocervix with 6–50% of solid growth pattern. Staging for endometrial cancer is as follows:

Stage I	Confined to uterine corpus
Ia	Limited to endometrium
Ib	Invades < 50% of the myometrium
Ic	Invades > 50% of the myometrium
Stage II	Involves the uterine corpus and cervix
IIa	Limited to endocervix
IIb	Invades cervical stroma
Stage III	Regional tumor spread to the pelvis
IIIa	Invades serosa and/or adnexa and/or malignant cells in peritoneal cytology
IIIb	Vaginal metastases
IIIc	Metastases to pelvic and/or paraaortic lymph nodes
Stage IV	Advanced pelvic disease or distant metastases
IVa	Invades bladder and/or bowel mucosa
IVb	Distant metastases (upper abdomen, inguinal lymph nodes, supraclavicular lymph nodes, lungs, liver, bones, brain)

Each stage of disease is evaluated for the degree of cellular differentiation and assigned a grade. The grading system is based primarily on the architectural findings, which are described by the percentage of solid tumor growth.

Grade 1	5% or less of a solid growth pattern
Grade 2	6–50% of a solid growth pattern
Grade 3	>50% of a solid growth pattern

8 The most appropriate primary surgery for this patient is

A. TAH-BSO

B. (MD Anderson) type II radical hysterectomy with pelvic and paraaortic lymph node sampling/dissection (P&PA-LNS)

C. (MD Anderson) type III radical hysterectomy with omentectomy and lymph node sampling

D. TAH-BSO, peritoneal washings, pelvic and paraaortic lymph node sampling (P&PA-LNS), and omentectomy

B MD Anderson type II radical hysterectomy with pelvic and paraaortic lymph node sampling/dissection (P&PA-LNS/D): this involves the resection of the cardinal ligaments flush with the pelvic side wall, the uterosacral ligaments well posteriorly and lateral to the rectum, and a 2–3-cm cuff of vagina. This surgery offers the best prognosis for disease of this stage.

9 The 5-year survival rate based on the initial stage of her disease is

A. 66%

B. 44%

C. 16%

D. 86%

E. Less than 5%

A Five-year survival rates are as follows: stage I, 86%; stage II, 66%; stage III, 44%; and stage IV, 16%. In addition, within a given stage of disease, a variety of clinical and histologic factors serve as additional prognostic variables, e.g., depth of myometrial invasion, malignancy of peritoneal washings, histologic grade and type, DNA ploidy, lymphatic space invasion, tumor bulk, estrogen and progesterone receptors, and patient age.

45

Ovarian Cancer

Amer Karam

1 A 56-year-old woman, gravida 3, para 2012, presents for her annual exam. She expresses concerns about ovarian cancer, as her next-door neighbor recently succumbed to the disease. She reports that her maternal grandmother succumbed to breast cancer and that one of her uncles died of lung cancer. The appropriate evaluation for this patient should include:

A. A CA-125 level

B. Screening for BRCA1/BRCA2

C. A rectovaginal examination

D. A transvaginal ultrasound

E. A pelvic MRI

C Current recommendations for screening include a comprehensive family history and annual rectovaginal pelvic examination for women with no significant family history of ovarian cancer. Women with two or more first-degree relatives with ovarian cancer have a 3% chance of having a familial ovarian cancer syndrome, which carries a 40% lifetime risk of ovarian cancer; these women should be examined and counseled by a gynecologic oncologist. Women with a familial ovarian cancer syndrome should undergo annual recto vaginal pelvic examination, CA-125 determination, and transvaginal ultrasonography.

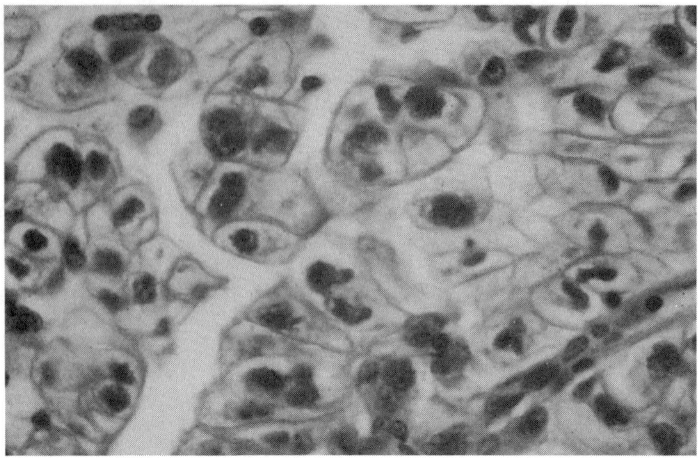

FIGURE 45.1 Surgical frozen specimen.

2 A 54-year-old woman, gravida 1, para 1001, is undergoing an exploratory laparotomy for an adnexal mass. The frozen section is shown in Figure 45.1. She reports a recent history of fevers and a remote history of endometriosis. The most likely pathologic diagnosis is

A. A serous tumor
B. A mucinous tumor
C. A dysgerminoma
D. A clear cell tumor
E. An endometroid tumor

D Clear cell carcinomas account for 3% of ovarian cancers. Histologically, hobnail-shaped cells are characteristic of clear cell carcinomas. These tumors are the ovarian neoplasms most commonly associated with paraneoplastic syndromes, including hypercalcemia and hyperpyrexia. The mean age at diagnosis is 53 years. Bilaterality occurs in 13% of cases. Clear cell carcinomas also have been associated with endometrial cancer and endometriosis.

3 A 49-year-old, gravida 3, para 3003, underwent primary cytoreductive surgery for stage IIIC ovarian carcinoma, with the largest remaining nodule measuring 3 cm. She received 6

cycles of carboplatin and Taxol chemotherapy postoperatively. The most important factor affecting her outcome is

A. Her initial response to chemotherapy
B. The size of the residual disease
C. Her Kamofsky index
D. Her family history
E. Her preoperative CA-125 level

B Primary cytoreductive surgery, or debulking, is the most important treatment of advanced disease. No universal agreement on the precise definition of optimal debulking has been reached. Different authors use different definitions of "optimal" in their measures of residual disease; these values range from 1 to 2 cm. The measurement of residual disease does not include the total volume of tumor cells left behind but merely the diameter of the largest residual nodule. Aggressive attempts at cytoreduction have been shown to improve long-term survival.

4 A 63-year-old woman, gravida 1, para 0010, underwent an exploratory laparotomy, washings, total abdominal hysterectomy, bilateral salpingo-oophorectomy, infracolic omentectomy, peritoneal and lymph node biopsies. The final pathology revealed a grade I serous adenocarcinoma involving both ovaries. All other pathologic biopsies were negative for tumor. The next step in her management should be

A. Intraperitoneal cisplatin
B. Taxol and carboplatin chemotherapy
C. Close monitoring with CA-125 levels
D. Whole abdominal irradiation
E. Second-look laparotomy in 6 months

C Patients with stage IA or IB disease and with grade 1 tumors are considered to have a favorable prognosis, with a 5-year survival of 94–96%. Patients with moderately or poorly differentiated tumors of any stage, stage IC disease, or stage II disease are considered to have an unfavorable prognosis. For patients with early stage disease and favorable prognostic factors, no chemotherapy is indicated. After the procedure, the woman should be followed closely with pelvic examinations and CA-125 measurements.

5 A 68-year-old, gravida 3, para 3003, with a history of stage IIIC ovarian cancer presents with a 2-day history of progressive nausea and bilious emesis. Abdominal X-ray is consistent with a small bowel obstruction. The next step in her management should be

A. Surgical exploration
B. Placement of a nasogastric tube and intravenous hydration
C. Salvage chemotherapy
D. Whole abdominal irradiation
E. Placement of a percutaneous gastric tube

B Many women with ovarian cancer develop intestinal obstruction, either at initial diagnosis or with recurrent disease. Obstruction may be related to mechanical blockage or carcinomatous ileus. Correction of intestinal obstruction at initial treatment is usually possible; obstruction associated with recurrent disease, however, is a complex problem. Some of these obstructions may be treated conservatively with intravenous hydration, total parenteral nutrition, and gastric decompression. The decision to proceed with palliative surgery must be based on the physical condition of the patient and her expected survival. If patients are unable to undergo surgery or are judged to be poor operative candidates, placement of a percutaneous gastric tube may offer some relief.

6 A 37-year-old, gravida 2, para 2, presents with a 3-month history of progressive abdominal pain and distention as well as intermenstrual bleeding. The transvaginal ultrasound discloses a 12-cm right adnexal mass. On surgical exploration, frozen section reveals a granulosa cell tumor. Fertility-preserving treatment should include:

A. A contralateral ovarian wedge biopsy
B. Dilatation and curettage
C. An oophoropexy

D. Adjuvant chemotherapy

E. Abdominal irradiation

B The granulosa cell tumor is the most common malignant sex cord stromal tumor. Granulosa cell tumors account for 2–3% of all ovarian malignancies. In the majority of cases, the tumor is estrogenic. Patients may present with abdominal distention, pain, or a mass. Because most granulosa cell tumors produce estrogen, patients may present with a variety of menstrual irregularities. The incidence of concurrent endometrial hyperplasia is 50%, and the incidence of concurrent endometrial adenocarcinoma is at least 5%. The majority of affected patients present with stage I disease, mainly because the hormonal effects of the tumor cause symptoms early in the disease. Surgery alone is usually sufficient treatment only for disease of stage IA or IB. If the patient desires to maintain fertility, a unilateral salpingo-oophorectomy is adequate for treating stage IA tumors, and a staging operation also should be perfomed. If the patient has completed her childbearing, a total abdominal hysterectomy and bilateral salpingo-oophorectomy should be performed. If the uterus is left *in situ,* dilation and curettage should be performed to rule out endometrial hyperplasia or adenocarcinoma. Chemotherapy after surgery does not prevent recurrence of the disease, which may occur late (10–15 years after diagnosis).

46

Gestational Trophoblastic Disease

Javier Soto

1 A 21-year-old patient underwent evacuation of a hydatidiform mole at 12 weeks' gestation without major complications. At the moment of evacuation her chest radiograph showed no evidence of pulmonary disease. The most appropriate follow-up for this patient is

A. Repeat chest radiograph 2 weeks after evacuation

B. Daily measurement of serum B-hCG levels until normal

C. Measurement of serum B-hCG levels 48 hours after evacuation and then monthly thereafter for 6–12 consecutive months

D. Measurement of serum B-hCG levels 48 hours after evacuation, weekly thereafter until results are normal for 3 consecutive weeks, and then monthly for 6–12 consecutive months

D Once the diagnosis of a hydatidiform mole has been made, the primary treatment is suction dilation and curettage (D&C). Preoperative workup should include hematologic studies (CBC), coagulation studies (PT, aPTT), blood chemistry and liver function tests, blood type and screen, quantitative B-hCG level, and chest radiograph. Twenty percent of evacuated complete moles are followed by persistent gestational trophoblastic disease. For this reason, patients should be carefully followed for early detection. Appropriate follow-up includes measurement of serum B-hCG levels 48 hours after evacuation, weekly thereafter until results are normal for 3 consecutive weeks, and then monthly for 6–12 consecutive months. Pelvic examinations should be performed to monitor the involution of pelvic organs and to evaluate for metastasis. Repeat chest radiograph is indicated only if there is a plateau or rise in B-hCG levels. In order to avoid confusion with a new pregnancy, appropriate contraception should be utilized throughout the follow-up period.

2 A 32-year-old woman underwent evacuation of a complete hydatidiform mole 2 months ago without complication. Preoperative evaluation (CBC, PT, aPTT, blood chemistry, and liver function test) was within normal limits. Her blood type is O positive. Chest radiograph showed no evidence of pulmonary disease. Quantitative B-hCG level at the time of evacuation was 150,000 mIU/mL. Her quantitative B-hCG levels have been followed weekly since evacuation. For the last 3 weeks her B-hCG levels have been increasing: 132,000 mIU/mL, 230,000 mIU/mL, and 758,000 mIU/mL. The patient has been on oral contraceptive pill therapy since evacuation. Repeat chest radiograph, and computerized tomography (CT) scans of the abdomen, pelvis, and brain were all normal, as were repeat CBC, liver function tests, thyroid function tests, and renal function tests. Ultrasound evaluation of the pelvis showed no evidence of intrauterine pregnancy. The most appropriate treatment for this patient is

A. Continue to follow B-hCG levels

B. Single-agent chemotherapy with actinomycin-D or methotrexate sodium

C. Combination chemotherapy with etoposide, methotrexate, actinomycin-D, cyclophosphamide, and vincristine sulfate

D. Hysterectomy and combination chemotherapy

B Twenty percent of evacuated complete moles are followed by persistent gestational trophoblastic disease (GTD). Persistent GTD includes invasive mole, choriocarcinoma, and placental site trophoblastic tumor (PSTT). The diagnosis of persistent GTD is most often made by a plateau or rise in B-hCG titers observed during follow-up of hydatidiform mole. It may also present with signs and symptoms related to metastatic disease, i.e., shortness of breath or chest pain with pulmonary metastasis. After diagnosis of persistent GTD has been made, appropriate workup to evaluate extent of disease and evaluate for possible metastases should take place. This workup should include thyroid, liver, and renal function tests; CBC; chest radiograph; CT of the pelvis, abdomen, and brain; pelvic ultrasonography; and stool guaiac test.

Treatment of persistent GTD is based on the presence of risk factors for treatment failure and on extent of disease. Low risk factors include short duration of disease (less than 4 months), serum B-hCG levels of 40,000 mIU/mL or less, no evidence of brain or liver metastases, no antecedent term pregnancy, and no prior chemotherapy. High risk factors include long duration of disease (longer than 4 months), serum B-hCG of greater than 40,000 mIU/mL, brain or liver metastases, antecedent term pregnancy, and prior chemotherapy. For nonmetastatic or low-risk disease the recommended primary therapy is single-agent chemotherapy with either methotrexate sodium or actinomycin-D. For patients with high-risk, metastatic disease the mainstay treatment consists of combination chemotherapy with etoposide, methotrexate, actinomycin-D, cyclophosphamide, and vincristine sulfate. Hysterectomy is reserved for patients with large intrauterine tumor burden, intrauterine infection, uterine hemorrhage, or patients who have failed single-agent chemotherapy.

3 A 19-year-old patient presents for her first prenatal visit with complaints of having two episodes of postcoital bleeding. According to her last menstrual period, she is in her 11th week of gestation. Vaginal examination reveals a closed cervix without evidence of bleeding. Her uterine size is consistent with a 20-week-sized gestation. Serum B-hCG level is 250,000 mIU/mL. Ultrasound evaluation reveals no evidence of a fetus and presence of cystic structures within the uterus with a snowstorm appearance. After evacuation of the complete mole chromosome analyses will most likely show

A. 46,XX

B. 69,XXY

C. 46,YY

D. 69,XXX

A Complete moles are usually diploid with a 46,XX karyotype. The chromosomal complements are usually paternally derived as a result of duplication of a haploid sperm pronucleus after fertilization of an empty ovum. Unlike complete moles, incomplete or partial moles are triploid, with two paternal sets and a maternal chromosome complement. The most common chromosomal complement is 69,XXY, seen in about 70% of cases. These are believed to arise from fertilization of an egg with a haploid set of chromosomes, either by two sperm or by a diploid sperm.

47

Chemotherapy and Radiation Therapy

Patricia Moore

1 A 49-year-old woman presents with complaints of bloating and increasing abdominal girth. On pelvic exam she is found to have a large pelvic mass. Abdominal computerized tomography (CT) scan reveals evidence of a 10 × 8 × 6 cm complex pelvic mass, omental caking, 1 × 1 cm liver metastasis, and enlarged paraaortic lymph nodes. Decision is made to treat with three cycles of carboplatin and paclitaxel before proceeding with debulking surgery. This is an example of

A. Primary chemotherapy

B. Neoadjuvant chemotherapy

C. Adjuvant chemotherapy

D. Salvage chemotherapy

B This patient is receiving chemotherapy in hopes of shrinking her tumor burden before she undergoes debulking surgery. This is neoadjuvant chemotherapy. After her optimal debulking surgery she will need further cycles of chemotherapy. This will be adjuvant chemotherapy. If that chemotherapy ultimately fails and she has disease recurrence needing additional chemotherapy, that will be salvage chemotherapy. Primary chemotherapy means using chemotherapy as the sole treatment for the disease process, such as in leukemia.

2 A 60-year-old woman has a history of stage IIIc ovarian cancer. In the past she has been treated with carboplatin, paclitaxel, ifosfamide, and doxorubicin. She develops progressive dyspnea on exertion, paroxysmal nocturnal dyspnea, and fatigue. Echocardiogram shows evidence of a dilated cardiomyopathy and congestive heart failure. The chemotherapeutic agent most likely responsible for this is

A. Carboplatin

B. Paclitaxel

C. Ifosfamide

D. Doxorubicin

D One of the known side effects of doxorubicin is cardiotoxicity resulting in irreversible cardiomyopathies leading to congestive heart failure, pleural effusions, dilated heart, and venous congestion. The effect is cumulative and thus careful attention must be paid to the cumulative dose of doxorubicin given to a patient. It is also prudent to obtain a baseline ejection fraction on a patient before starting these agents. Other common side effects associated with doxorubicin include myelosuppression, alopecia, mucosal ulcerations, and nausea and vomiting.

Paclitaxel has also been known to cause cardiac side effects. However, these are more commonly transient signs or symptoms such as bradycardia, ventricular tachycardia, and chest pain, and tend to resolve with slowing of the infusion rate. It is also associated with myelosuppression, alopecia, and allergic reactions.

The common side effects associated with carboplatin are neuropathy, nephrotoxicity, ototoxicity, and myelosuppresion. Cisplatin has a similar profile but with more neuropathy, nephrotoxicity, and ototoxicity but less myelosuppression.

Ifosfamide is associated with myelosuppression, hemorrhagic cystitis, CNS dysfunction, and nephrotoxicity. In order to prevent hemorrhagic cystitis, mesna is given with ifosfamide and cyclophosphamide. Mesna protects the bladder by neutralizing acrolein, the metabolite responsible for the bladder toxicity.

3 A 64-year-old woman has undergone optimal debulking surgery for stage IIIa ovarian cancer. During her hospital stay she undergoes her first cycle of chemotherapy with carboplatin and paclitaxel. During the paclitaxel infusion you are called to see her. She tells you her abdomen is hurting and she feels sweaty. She appears flushed. Her pulse is 50 and her blood pressure is 90/50. After stopping the infusion you give her diphenhydramine, dexamethasone, and ranitidine. You then tell her:

A. She is allergic to paclitaxel, and you will need to choose a new chemotherapeutic agent for her.

B. She is allergic to cremaphor, the vehicle used to administer paclitaxel, and you will need to choose a different chemotherapeutic agent for her.

C. She will need a slower infusion rate of paclitaxel to prevent this reaction in the future.

D. This is a common hypersensitivity reaction to cremaphor, the vehicle used to administer paclitaxel, and in the future she will need to be pretreated with diphenhydramine, dexamethasone, and ranitidine before each dose of paclitaxel.

D Paclitaxel is made from the western yew tree. It is insoluble and thus cremaphor is used as a vehicle for its administration. Unfortunately, approximately 1% of patients have a hypersensitivity reaction to the cremaphor. Thus, these people need to be pretreated with steroids as well as histamine-1 and histamine-2 blockers. These people then tend to tolerate the infusion very well. Slowing of the infusion rate alone will not solve the problem. However, there is no need to abandon the use of paclitaxel in these patients.

4 A 53-year-old woman is undergoing teletherapy or external-beam radiation therapy for vaginal cancer. After her third week of treatment she presents to you complaining of a rash appearing in the perineal and inguinal regions. She complains of pruritus and erythema with desquamation. You may tell her all of the following *except:*

A. Use topical corticosteroids and moisturizers.

B. Explain that these reactions usually clear up 3 weeks after treatment ends.

C. Tell her that treatment may need to be stopped temporarily if the reaction worsens, in order to treat the area with zinc oxide or silver sulfadiazine and to allow it to heal.

D. This is a rare reaction and you will refer her to a dermatologist immediately.

D This acute skin reaction to radiation therapy is very common. Usually it can be treated with topical corticosteroids and moisturizers. Once the radiation therapy is completed, it should resolve. However, some patients may need to stop treatments in order to allow the skin to heal before completing their therapy.

5 A 33-year-old woman presents to you after starting external-beam radiation therapy for cervical cancer. She says that a few hours after her first treatment she developed nausea, vomiting, and diarrhea, which has continued ever since. You tell her:

A. She most likely has viral gastroenteritis.

B. She is having a common reaction to radiation therapy and it will improve with time.

C. She is having a common reaction to radiation therapy, and she should take loperamide for relief of her diarrhea and antiemetics for her nausea.

D. She has reached the maximum dose of radiation her bowel can withstand, and all further therapy must be halted.

C Acute gastrointestinal complications are common. They usually occur 2–6 hours after abdominal or pelvic irradiation. The treatment for this complication includes hydration, antiemetics, and antidiarrheals. Loperamide is usually the first-choice antidiarrheal, followed by diphenoxylate. If those fail to work, then tincture of opium, paregoric, or codeine may be used. For high-output diarrhea, octreotide can help as well.

48

Palliative Care

Dana Virgo

Please read the following vignette to answer Questions 1 and 2.
A 42-year-old woman with metastatic breast cancer with progressive peritoneal carcinomatosis and symptoms of intractable nausea, vomiting, and worsening ascites is admitted for intraperitoneal catheter placement for drainage of ascites and administration of intraperitoneal chemotherapy. She does not have an advance directive and has not discussed her code status with her oncologist.

---

1 As the admitting physician, you:

A. Wait for the patient and her family to bring up advance care planning as a sign that they are ready to discuss it.

B. Counsel the patient on choosing her code status and recommend that she formulate an advance directive with the assistance of her family.

C. Recommend that the patient discuss advance care planning with her oncologist as an outpatient.

B Advance care planning is the process of discussing end-of-life care, involving the explicit formulation and recording of the patient's wishes. The Federal Patient Self-Determination Act requires health care institutions participating in Medicare and Medicaid programs to inform all adult patients of their rights to make decisions concerning their care and to formulate advance directives. The existence of advance directives must be noted in the patient's chart. The importance of advance planning from a psychosocial as well as legal and ethical standpoints cannot be overemphasized. Nonetheless, only about 20% of hospitalized patients have advance directives.

Ideally, advance care planning is initiated early in the patient–physician relationship so that the patient, family and caregivers, and the treating physician have ample time to consider all options. However, many physicians hesitate to initiate discussions of advance planning because of concerns about upsetting patients, as well as unfamiliarity and discomfort with the issues involved. Physicians may feel that addressing end-of-life issues will undermine the therapeutic intent of treatment or take away patient hope. However, evidence shows that most patients believe that their physicians should initiate discussion of advance care planning. Thought and discussion about the issues involved are important components of patient adaptation to chronic or life-threatening illness. Patients may find it helpful to discuss advance care planning with multiple members of the health care team, including nursing staff and social workers. Patients may be fearful of the reaction of family and friends to a frank discussion about end-of-life care. Even healthy patients should be encouraged to discuss the important issues of advance planning with their families and consider their wishes in the event of sudden incapacitation. This discussion, especially in the context of serious illness, should include the issue of code status. It also should include creating an advance directive, oral or written instructions about future medical care in the event the individual is unable to communicate. The patient may choose to select a family member or a friend to hold health care power of attorney as well.

Advance care planning is best discussed with patients and their families by providers who know them well. However, if these issues are not discussed or resolved, the resident physician or hospitalist caring for the patient acutely cannot neglect them.

2 The patient maintains full code status, declines to formulate an advance care directive, and chooses her husband as her decision maker in the event that she is incapacitated. Soon after admission, she is transferred to the intensive care unit with sepsis and respiratory failure requiring intubation and pressor support. Her condition worsens despite multiple invasive interventions. The medical team caring for the patient counsels her husband that her prognosis is extremely poor, and recommends comfort care measures without continued aggressive treatment. Her husband strongly states his desire to pursue all available treatment. The team requests an ethics consult. As a member of the hospital ethics committee, you recommend:

A. That further aggressive management be withheld due to the futility of the situation

B. That a family conference be held to facilitate further decision making about her care

C. That the patient's husband, in his capacity holding health care power of attorney, should continue to make decisions for the patient

C The importance of informed consent rests on the assumption of patient autonomy. Autonomy, implies noninterference in decision making by others. The right of patients to refuse medical treatment has been affirmed by the U.S. Supreme Court. The physician's ethical obligation is to respect patient autonomy while observing beneficence, the obligation to do good, as well as its corollary, nonmaleficence, or doing no harm. In this case, medical decision making by the team is a difficult balance between patient autonomy and beneficence, since the wishes of the designated health care decision maker do not agree with the physicians' recommendations, which were formulated to optimize outcome and minimize harm. In the context of terminal illness, there is no legal or societal consensus for situations in which patients and families disagree with physicians' recommendations to stop treatment. In general, the right of patients to request treatment considered futile or inappropriate has been observed by the medical community.

When a patient is incapacitated and cannot make decisions, the wishes expressed by her advance directive or by the person designated to have health care power of attorney are respected, again due to the importance of patient autonomy. In circumstances where the medical team and the patient or the patient's representative differ with regard to level of care, maintenaince of an open, ongoing, nonconfrontational dialogue is essential.

Please read the following vignette to answer Questions 3 and 4.

A 52-year-old woman with recurrent stage IIIB squamous cell carcinoma of the cervix has undergone whole pelvic radiation therapy and brachytherapy with cisplatin chemosensitization, now has recurrence of her disease in her periaortic and iliac nodes and is undergoing salvage chemotherapy. The patient has a remote history of narcotic abuse, and adequate pain control has been a chronic problem. She presents to the office complaining of severe, chronic pain. She also complains of decreased appetite, fatigue, and lack of energy, and is frequently tearful during her visit. She is on an analgesic regimen of controlled-release oxycodone 100 mg twice daily with Tylox (oxycodone 5 mg/acetaminophen 325 mg) as needed for break-through pain. The patient estimates that she takes at least 15 tablets of Tylox daily.

---

3 The *best* strategy for managing this patient's pain is

A. Consulting social work and the hospital's chronic pain service for this patient's persistent narcotic addiction.

B. Prescribing a selective serotonin reuptake inhibitor (SSRI) for her depression.

C. Increasing her dose of oxycodone, adding celecoxib (Celebrex), and changing her regimen for break-through pain to morphine.

D. Discussion of enrollment in a hospice program.

C Adequate pain relief in seriously ill patients is a challenge, particularly when the patient has a history of narcotic abuse. Tolerance to narcotics will develop in any patient on narcotic medications over time, and even patients with stable disease may require increasing doses of narcotics to control their pain. Narcotic tolerance does not necessarily mean that narcotic addiction is present. In general, the risk of addiction in the setting of terminal disease is minimal. In this particular patient, increasing the dose of her long-acting narcotic and adding an adjuvant drug, in this case a nonsteroidal antiinflammatory drug, should better control her pain without requiring her to take large amounts of Tylox. Due to the acetominophen component of Tylox and the patient's history of overadministration of Tylox, it would be prudent to change her break-through regimen to morphine or another non-acetaminophen-containing short-acting narcotic.

Chronically or terminally ill patients with a history of substance abuse should not be punished for their history by withholding of appropriate pain management. This particular patient likely would benefit from assessment by the chronic pain service to help manage her chronic severe pain. She also would benefit from continued social work follow-up for assessment of lingering substance abuse issues, grief and depression, coping skills, etc. Patients with recurrent cancer and poorly controlled pain have a high risk for depression. Addition of an SSRI or a tricyclic antidepressant (TCA) would not only target this patient's depression, but might also improve her pain control. An antidepressant would supplement her narcotics regimen, not replace adequate narcotic treatment, however.

Most hospice programs require patients to have a prognosis of no longer than 6 months of life. This particular patient continues to receive chemotherapy, which also is prohibited by most hospice programs. An in-depth discussion of short- and long-term goals for treatment, including curative versus palliative therapy, pain control, and advance planning, is recommended periodically in oncology patients, with hospice being considered as needed.

4 What regimen would be most appropriate to prevent constipation in this patient?

A. Constipation should not be a problem in this patient because of her narcotics tolerance.

B. Treat with cathartic or osmotic laxatives as necessary.

C. Start a prophylactic regimen including increasing exercise and fluid intake, increasing dietary fiber, and osmotic laxatives.

C Constipation is a major problem in terminally ill patients and in those on narcotic pain medications. Most patients develop tolerance to the narcotic side effects of nausea and pruritus, but not to constipation. A prophylactic approach to constipation is most effective.

General recommendations include regular exercise, when possible. Increasing fluid intake to at least 1.5 L daily may be helpful. Increasing dietary fiber to increase stool bulk and water content is also helpful. This may be accomplished inexpensively using bran powder; alternatively, fiber supplements such as psyllim or methylcellulose may be used. Notably, fluid intake must be adequate for fiber supplements to be effective.

Prophylactic pharmacologic therapy may include osmotic laxatives, saline laxatives, emollient laxatives, nonabsorbable sugars, and cisapride. Osmotic laxatives soften stools without inducing dependency. They are titrated to a dose that results in soft to semiliquid stools.

Index